BACK AND NECK PAIN

A COMPLETE PLAN FOR SELF-DIAGNOSIS AND TREATMENT

ANDREW FERGUSON MRO

Pelham Books

Designed and produced by
Breslich & Foss
Golden House
28–31 Great Pulteney Street
London W1R 3DD

Editor: Jim Abram
Designer: Roger Daniels
Illustrations: Sheila Tizzard
Paste-up artist: Richard Slater
Editorial: Judy Martin

First published in Great Britain by
Pelham Books Ltd
27 Wrights Lane
London W8 5TZ
1988

British Library Cataloguing in Publication Data

Ferguson, Andrew
    Back and neck pain: a complete plan
    for self-diagnosis and treatment.
    1. Backache —— Treatment
    I. Title
    616.7'3068   RD768

    ISBN 0-7207-1766-3

Typesetting by AKM Associates (UK) Ltd,
London
Printed and bound in Spain by Sirven Grafic, Barcelona

Contents

Introduction

Back and neck pain is one of the most frequent causes of discomfort and distress in our society; men and women of all ages suffer from it and it is responsible for many lost working days each year. Despite this, the diagnosis, treatment and prevention of back and neck pain is often inadequate, confusing and occasionally even harmful. A broad consideration of the person as a whole is often obscured by a narrow search for certain pathological diseases which might cause back and neck pain.

This book is based on the principles of holistic medicine, where all aspects of a person's health and lifestyle are taken into consideration. Increasing awareness of the relationship between the mind and body is encouraging a healthy scepticism towards some of the traditional attitudes to medical care: patients should not have to live with back and neck pain; doctors should not have to rely solely on drugs and surgery for treatment.

A central theme of this book is the role of muscular tension as a source of back and neck pain. This has been overlooked by many books on the subject, with the result that much effort has been wasted in the search for mythical 'slipped discs', and no time spent trying to uncover the real causes. One important cause of muscular tension is emotional tension; to acknowledge this psychosomatic link is a major step towards effective diagnosis and treatment. Each person's tensions are unique; it is only the individual who can, and should, take full responsibility for his or her own health.

The aim of this book is to help you to understand, resolve and prevent your own individual back and neck problem. I have presented a simple, coherent system for accurately diagnosing the various possible causes of back and neck pain, which means that your treatment can be more effective. The subject is covered thoroughly and in depth, but I have kept the reader constantly in mind – this is not a textbook full of unnecessary information. I hope that the book will be comprehensible to all as a result and that all will be able to benefit from it – health professional and lay reader alike.

A.F.

How Your Spine Works

*T*his chapter provides the background to a better understanding of your back or neck pain. Some of the facts and ideas outlined here may not seem immediately relevant and may even be superfluous for straightforward cases. In chronic or complicated cases, however, it will be necessary for you to take them into account, if you wish to diagnose and treat your problem successfully.

Anatomy

The Spine

The spine connects the head to the pelvic bones and supports the rib cage. It is made up of smaller units of bone called vertebrae, which get progressively smaller higher up the spine, as they bear less body weight. The vertebrae are connected by discs, muscles and ligaments, and there are joints between them which enable them to move in relation to each other. It is this movement between the vertebrae that gives the spine its flexibility.

The column formed by the vertebrae also encloses and protects the spinal cord and the nerves that run to and from it, connecting the brain with the rest of the body.

The spine is divided into five areas:

1 Cervical or neck area, made up of seven vertebrae.

2 Thoracic or mid back area, made up of twelve vertebrae.

3 Lumbar or low back area, made up of five vertebrae.

4 Sacrum, five vertebrae fused together to form one bone that joins the pelvic bones.

5 Coccyx, four very small vertebrae fused together; this is the non-functioning remains of a tail.

Neck Area The neck is adapted to meet the demands of the special senses of vision, hearing and balance. It is very mobile and able to move in all directions, yet it is also capable of very fine adjustments, such as keeping the eyes level and facing forwards. This is due to the fact that the shape of the upper two vertebrae is different from the others and they are surrounded by many small muscles to finely control their position.

Thoracic Area There are twelve ribs on each side of the spine, which protect the contents of the thorax and aid breathing. They also limit overall mobility; unlike the low back and neck areas the thorax is not designed for a great range of movement.

The Spine, Vertebrae and Discs

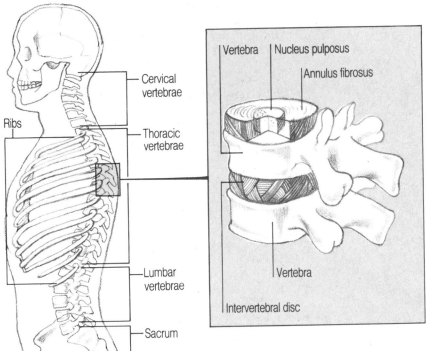

Cervical vertebrae

Ribs

Thoracic vertebrae

Vertebra | Nucleus pulposus

Annulus fibrosus

Lumbar vertebrae

Vertebra

Intervertebral disc

Sacrum

Coccyx

The central pillar of your skeleton is the spine, formed from blocks of bone called vertebrae. The front of each vertebra is a strong cylinder of bone to bear the weight of the body. Sandwiched between these are the discs, which are strong, yet flexible enough to allow movement.

At the rear of the vertebrae are projections of bone. Attached to these are strong muscles and ligaments, which protect the spine and control movement. Each vertebra has a hollow circle of bone in the middle and the vertical alignment of the vertebrae forms a canal through which the spinal cord passes. There are four smooth surfaces, or facets, on the rear projections of bone, two above and two below, which form joints with the vertebrae immediately above and below.

Low Back Area   The low back area is under most strain, as it has to bear the weight of the whole of the upper body and be able to perform bending and twisting movements.

The sacrum, the pelvic bones and the coccyx form the skeleton of the pelvis, which is not designed for a great deal of movement.

Vertebrae

The vertebrae (bones) are dense and strong structures made principally of calcium and other minerals. Bone is a relatively inert tissue and does not change very quickly, although one musn't forget that it is living and not dead. Due to this there are few things that can go wrong with them; occasionally a vertebra develops in an unusual shape, or it may be affected by specific conditions associated with childhood and old age. Diseases of the bone are very rare. In bad infections such as tuberculosis, or in advanced cancer, the disease may spread to the bones, but the widespread symptoms and effects of these conditions will usually be the major problems rather than back or neck pain.

The conditions most frequently seen in the vertebrae themselves are degenerative changes and, less commonly, fractures.

Discs

The discs are very strong, yet are capable of a degree of compression and deformation, which allows movement to occur between the vertebrae. Discs are made of a jelly-like centre, called the nucleus pulposus, surrounded by layers of tough fibrous tissue and cartilage, called the annulus fibrosus. This material has no nerve or blood supply, which means that the discs are not sensitive to pain. If they are damaged they take a long time to heal.

As the discs are so strong it takes a lot to damage them; if a large force is suddenly applied to the spine the bones will fracture before the discs give way. What can damage the discs is repetitive strain over a period of time, usually many years, which means that disc problems are unlikely under the age of twenty.

Gradually the fibres in the annulus can tear and the softer material from the nucleus channels towards the surface of the disc. This not only contributes to degeneration of the disc but means that there is a possibility that the disc can bulge, or even herniate – which means that the nucleus leaks out of the disc. Once the disc has bulged it can press on nearby structures, such as the nerve roots and ligaments and cause symptoms. Due to the fact that it takes time and force to cause this damage, it is only likely to occur at the base of the spine in the lowest two discs; disc bulges or herniations elsewhere are rare.

All discs gradually change as you get older. From about the age of twenty the nucleus gradually becomes tougher. After about the age of fifty the nucleus is so tough that a herniation is virtually impossible. Another consequence of the changes in the disc is that it gets thinner with age and wear and tear; this is one of the factors that contributes to people losing body height in old age. These changes in the discs are called degenerative changes or spondylosis.

In summary, discs are strong structures and don't cause most of the problems that they are blamed for. Discs do not 'slip' out of place, nor can they be manipulated into place. Discs themselves are not pain-sensitive, but they may cause symptoms by affecting other structures.

Joints

Joints in the spine are similar in composition to joints elsewhere in your body, such as in your fingers. The bones are tipped by cartilage and are surrounded by a membrane, which secretes a lubricant called synovial fluid.

In the back and neck there are two small facet joints between each pair of vertebrae, one sacro-iliac joint each side of the sacrum, which join it to the pelvis, and joints between the ribs and the spine. In the spine the joints are well protected and rarely give trouble. However they can be involved in various forms of arthritis, which means 'joint inflammation'.

The joints may also be affected by trauma, especially in the neck and the sacro-iliac joints. If they are not kept flexible the surrounding tissues can shorten, decreasing the mobility of the joint and causing stiffness. This can put strain on the muscles of other areas, and can predispose to degenerative changes.

A condition known as 'locking' of spinal joints can occur, and is probably due to spasm in the small muscles immediately surrounding the joint.

Nerves

The spine encloses and protects the spinal cord which runs down the spinal canal from the brain. Nerves arise from the spinal cord and pass out between each pair of vertebrae. Once they have left the spine the nerves branch out and supply all the tissues in their area, particularly the muscles. They also receive information from the joints, skin, tendons and muscles.

Nerves are vulnerable to a number of conditions, such as lack of nutrients or poor circulation and rare diseases such as polio or multiple sclerosis. However the most frequent problem related to the back and neck is nerve irritation, caused by pressure on a nerve from another structure, such as discs or bones. Sometimes in the neck the spinal cord itself can be compressed.

Nerves usually recover if the irritation or compression is relieved, as long as it hasn't gone on for too long, but are less good at recovering from major physical damage or disease.

Ligaments

Ligaments are made of strong, usually inelastic, fibrous tissue. They hold bones together and prevent excessive movement. If the force applied to a ligament is too great, it can be overstretched and become inflamed, or in an extreme case it can be torn, though this is uncommon in the spine.

As the spine is relatively stable and well protected by muscles, problems in the ligaments are rare. The exception are the sacro-iliac ligaments and the ligaments in the neck, especially after trauma. Ligaments have a poor blood supply, so it often takes a few hours after an injury before they get inflamed. Once inflamed, however, they take a long time to heal.

The Nerves and Disc Herniation

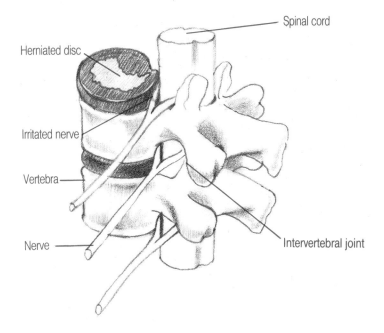

Spinal cord

Herniated disc

Irritated nerve

Vertebra

Nerve

Intervertebral joint

Nerves run out from the spinal cord through the small space on either side of the vertebra. They pass behind the discs and in front of the intervertebral joints. This arrangement means that the nerves can be irritated or compressed by anything that pushes against them, such as a bulging or herniated disc (above). This can also occur if the bone of the vertebra or joint enlarges due to degenerative changes.

When a nerve is irritated the effects can be felt along the length of the nerve. In cases in the low back, this can be all the way down to the foot. In the neck irritated nerves can cause symptoms in the arm or hand. The spinal cord itself is rarely irritated or compressed, except occasionally in the neck from advanced degenerative changes or after major trauma.

Muscles

Muscles are generally the most underestimated tissues when it comes to the assessment of back and neck problems. 'Slipped discs', 'trapped nerves', 'torn ligaments' and 'displaced bones' are often incorrectly blamed, but muscular problems are the cause of most cases of back or neck pain.

Muscles are the only tissues that can move the body. They can change rapidly; they surround and control the stability and position of all our tissues; they make up over forty per cent of the body and without them nothing would work. Even the heart and intestines are made of muscle.

The anatomical arrangement of the muscles is worth noting. They surround the front, back and sides of the whole body, and are formed in layers, each layer running in a different direction. Thus the trunk can be moved, controlled, and stabilized by the complicated and very fine coordination of all the muscle groups.

There are four states that a muscle can be in:

1   **Relaxed.** This is a healthy resting tone, as muscles are never totally inactive.

2   **Contracted.** When a muscle contracts it shuts down its own blood supply and drainage. Prolonged contraction causes an accumulation of waste chemicals, which can cause pain. Contraction is reversible.

3   **Fibrotic.** If a muscle is chronically contracted without adequate relaxation time, the lack of nutrition causes the laying down of fibrous tissue in some of the muscle. This gives badly used muscles a stringy, hard and tender feel. Fibrotic muscles ache easily after little use. Fibrosis can be eased by massage and exercise.

4   **In Spasm.** This is the name given when a muscle contracts forcefully, which can be extremely painful. Spasm can be a good reflex to splint and protect a damaged structure, or it can be inappropriate when the controlling nerves are functioning incorrectly.

Most muscles can be restored to good function with the self-help treatment methods outlined in this book, thus you can relieve most back and neck problems. Actual diseases affecting muscles are rare, and tearing of muscles is unusual, except occasionally in the limbs through common athletic injuries such as pulled hamstrings.

Basic Spinal Curves

From an evolutionary viewpoint, man evolved from walking on all four limbs to walking on hind limbs. This meant that the spine assumed a vertical orientation and over time it has evolved and adapted well to that position. Contrary to accepted opinion, the spine is well designed and can support you throughout your life, providing you use it and look after it well.

Looking at the spine from behind, it should ideally be straight. Many people, however, have a slightly asymmetrical curve, most commonly due to unequal leg lengths. The difference in length is usually about 0.5cm ($\frac{1}{4}$in), but it is not uncommon to have a difference of 1cm ($\frac{1}{2}$in) or more. The body can usually cope with this situation well, by curving the spine to compensate for the difference. Most people are unaware that they have such curves, but they can act as predisposing factors to problems later on.

Looking at the spine from the side (see p.9) you will see a long forward curve in the thoracic area (called a kyphosis) with a backward curve in the cervical and lumbar areas (called a lordosis). This S-shaped curve is natural and allows more flexibility than a ramrod-straight spine would.

Not everyone's spinal shape is ideal and getting an idea of your own curves is useful. Posture is a result of the interaction of a number of complex, highly individual influences, which are covered in Chapter Two – Take Your Personal Case History. Once established your basic posture will be difficult to alter without changing some long-standing attitudes and patterns of tension, but it can be improved by the exercises outlined in the section on Posture (p.121).

It is extremely important that you work to improve your posture, as correct posture will decrease the amount of work your muscles have to do to keep you upright. This will in turn help to decrease tension in the back muscles.

Movement and Control

Movement

Even when we are asleep or resting the body is always active in varying degrees. Thus it is important to understand the dynamics of movement and particularly what controls, coordinates and influences it. When a problem arises you will then have a better idea of the causes and what you can do about it.

Movement requires that all the tissues in the area of moving spine are in a healthy enough state to allow it:

■ The bones have to be able to support the changes in weight that pass through them.

■ The discs have to be strong enough to distort and be compressed without tearing, bulging or pressing on nearby tissues.

■ The ligaments have to be intact and not inflamed, so that they don't hurt at the end of the movement and can do their job of preventing the movement going too far.

■ The joint surfaces have to be able to slide on each other and the tissues around the joint must be free of inflammation, to allow pain-free motion.

■ The nerves have to be intact, to control the movement and there should be nothing that compresses or irritates them. If a disc, for example, is compressing a nerve, the nerve won't be able to slide freely; the movement will be painful and limited and will probably cause nerve symptoms, such as pins and needles or numbness in a leg or foot.

■ The muscles should be able to allow, control and balance the movement. This is a complicated demand as there are some muscles that have to lengthen to allow the movement, some that have to shorten to take up the slack, and some that have to work to balance you, so that you don't fall over or put strain on other structures. All the time they also have to counter the effects of gravity and do the work you require of them. In fact, most movement, and even staying in one position, involves the coordinated balance of most of your muscles, which is why controlling them is so important.

Local Control

Local control of the muscles is by automatic and involuntary reflexes. The spinal cord acts like a telephone exchange, coordinating the information received and producing the correct commands to do whatever is required. Each vertebra has a pair of nerves that pass beneath it, and these supply a given area of tissue; the nerves and vertebrae are called a segment and there are thirty-two such segments along the spine. Some of the segments also supply the heart, lungs, digestive tract, uterus, kidneys and sinuses, so disturbances in these tissues can affect the related segment of the spine and vice versa. This explains how pain and cramp in the colon or uterus can cause pain or muscular tension in the low back, and how rubbing or warming the skin can sometimes ease underlying muscular or visceral problems.

In response to pain or damage, the reflexes can increase the tension in the muscles of the affected area, or cause them to go into spasm; this causes more pain, which in turn can lead to more spasm. This is known as the pain-spasm-pain reflex, which can turn a mild problem into severe distress.

General Control

The brain receives information from the spinal cord and it can also influence it. The body works as a whole together with the mind, and any division into parts is artificial. Thus to understand the real cause of any problem you should not isolate one part and blame it, but rather consider yourself as a whole person. Your problem may be manifesting itself in a particular area, but it is likely to be a symptom of a more generalized disturbance. It is only by appreciating this combination of local and general influences that you can hope to resolve problems and improve your health.

Body Patterns Your body does not function by contracting individual muscles, but rather whole areas or movements. These can be thought of as your individual patterns of tension, which can be seen throughout your whole system. For example, you may have one side tighter than the other all the way down your body and you may get a headache or backache on that side more frequently than on the other. Further events such as trauma, scars and illnesses can alter these patterns.

Often patterns are superimposed or layered on top of each other, depending on the influences, so working them out and resolving them is sometimes difficult. These patterns may focus on one or two particular areas, which then tend to be the areas that are most vulnerable and the first to give symptoms under stress. Try to identify your own focuses or weak spots; they may be in any area of your body.

Stresses In addition to the patterns of muscular tension, there are chemical changes that can take place in the body and brain as a result of, for example, mood changes or nutritional imbalances – hormones come into this category. Influences such as illness, fatigue, trauma and shock can also affect your body as a whole.

These influences can be seen as stresses on your system, and can be broadly divided into mental, physical and chemical factors. They tend to add together, gradually reducing your ability to cope with further demands, until something goes and your health starts to suffer. Which part of you gives symptoms first depends on the individual focuses of tension mentioned above. Effects can vary from backache, indigestion or asthma to heart attack or mental breakdowns. Under stressful conditions you are vulnerable and more likely to develop back or neck pain.

Self-Image As the mind and body are part of one whole it is possible to view the body as the physical expression of the mind. This is readily apparent at a conscious or voluntary level: if you want to move your hand you can do so. Much control, however, occurs at a subconscious level of which you are not normally aware. Your subconscious self-image can therefore have a profound effect

18

on your body, for example:

- You may tense certain areas without realizing. In the pelvic area this may perhaps be due to anxiety about sexual matters.

- You may subconsciously reject an area, perhaps because it has hurt you, or you don't like it. This can block it off and stop it from healing or improving.

- You may feel unhappy or lacking in confidence at a deep level, causing you to tend to curl up and focus tension on your chest. This can contribute to breathing, digestive and heart problems.

- You may have a lot of bottled-up anger or strong feeling, which may show as jaw tension, teeth grinding or headaches. Individual patterns vary, but aggression is often associated with neck pain, fear with abdominal pain, and despair with low back pain.

These are just a few examples – each person has his or her own unique combination of influences. Wilhelm Reich called this control of emotions by muscular tension 'body armouring'. It has a protective function in blocking unpleasant feelings, but it also acts like a pressure cooker, causing the feelings to build up until something has to give.

Memory Memory is still not fully understood, but it does involve the body as well as the mind. A bad shock, for example, can cause a gasp, a contraction of the diaphragm and even temporary paralysis. After a while this shock may disappear, but unless it has been completely resolved, rather than pushed under the surface, some effects can still be found months, or even years, later in the body and mind, as unresolved events tend to accumulate.

It is a combination of mental health, emotional balance and physical well-being that enables us to carry on. Becoming aware of some of the patterns and subconscious focuses of tension can help you to become healthier. Learning to let go of tensions and to integrate rejected parts is a complex process and requires a lot of work and patience.

What Happens When Something Goes Wrong?

One of the first symptoms of a problem in the spine is pain. This can be useful to warn of damage or disease in your body, but in many cases, particularly if the pain is persistent or recurrent, the pain gives no benefit and can have severe adverse effects on the quality of your life.

Back and neck pains are no exception. A large percentage of people suffer such pain at some time in their lives and in many cases this can persist or recur over a number of years. As most back and neck pains are not due to serious diseases, there is often little to show on the surface how severe the pain actually is. This means that sufferers often get little sympathy from others, who may have only experienced minor twinges or passing aches.

The location where the pain is felt can occasionally vary as much as the severity with which it is felt. Pain arising from structures near the surface of the body is usually localized to the area affected. The deeper the structure causing the pain, the harder it is for the brain to tell exactly where it is coming from. In the case of very deep internal structures the pain can be 'referred' to somewhere else.

Referred Pain This is the name given to an experience of pain in a location other than the site of the structure causing the pain. It usually arises from disease or damage to internal organs, but can occur in some deep spinal problems related to the bones and discs. Examples of referred pain are heart pain felt across the front of the chest and down the left arm, and deep spinal pain felt down the leg (if from the low back) and in the arm (if from the neck). It is important to note here that referred spinal pain is unusual; leg and arm pains are usually due to local muscular tension.

Nerve Pain This is also variable and relatively uncommon. In cases of nerve irritation the degree of pain can range from none at all, to severe shooting pains along the course of the nerve. Nerve pain is unlikely in the absence of nerve symptoms such as pins and needles or numbness.

Take Your Personal Case History

This chapter is concerned with the important influences on you as an individual, with particular relevance to back and neck problems. Discovering the cause of your symptoms is not simply a case of giving the problem a name or label. You have to consider those factors at work on you as an individual that make your case different from any other.

Understanding Your Problem

To fully understand your problem you need to build up a 'diagnostic picture' of yourself, which includes past and present influences. This picture is wide-ranging, but it can be divided into three main areas:

1 Inherited factors.
2 Contributing factors, such as early influences, past events and general health.
3 Maintaining factors.

Once you have an understanding of these, the diagnosis of which tissues are causing your symptoms is more likely to be accurate in your particular case. In addition, when it comes to treatment, you will have a better idea of what you can do to improve the situation.

What follows is a list of the sort of questions that a good practitioner would ask you, together with a brief explanation as to why they may be important. You should consider your answers to these questions carefully and you might find it useful to write down any factors that you think are important in your case.

Inherited Factors

These are your genetic inheritance from your parents. Some inherited factors are only tendencies which may or may not be expressed in any particular case. For example, if there is rheumatoid arthritis in your family, the chances of you having it are greater than families which don't have it, but are nonetheless still quite small.

What are your overall build, proportions and height? The longer your spine the greater the leverage and strain there is on your back. If you have a narrow build, your spine is likely to be less strongly supported than that of someone who is broad-backed, thus tending to put more strain on your muscles and ligaments. If you are heavily built, your spine is likely to be stiffer and eventually more prone to degenerative changes than that of someone who is lightly built.

What are your soft tissues like?

If you are generally 'loose-limbed', with very mobile joints, you may be prone to joint or ligament strains and your muscles will have to work harder to hold you together. If you have generally solid or restricted joints, you are less likely to suffer joint strains, but you will be more prone to stiffness in the long-term.

Is there any condition that 'runs in the family'?

There are many conditions amongst blood relatives that show an inheritable tendency, ranging from diabetes to schizophrenia. Of particular importance in back and neck problems are family histories of rheumatoid arthritis and ankylosing spondylitis (see Arthritis p.146).

Have you any developmental anomalies that you know of?

Occasionally people are born with wrongly-formed vertebrae in various parts of the spine. Major anomalies can cause problems, but are rare (see Spinal Conditions p.147). The more common minor anomalies do not usually cause any problems and most people are unaware that they have them. Sometimes the anomaly can be as small as the angle of the joints at the base of the spine being slightly altered, which can put more stress on that area. You may have been told that you have this after having X-ray plates taken of your spine.

Early Influences

Did you have any difficulty in learning to crawl or walk as a baby?

Problems at this stage, for whatever reason, can cause incomplete development of many coordinative reflexes and possibly affect spinal curve development and posture. The development of basic reflexes has been linked with such diverse phenomena as dyslexia, not knowing left from right, visual problems, clumsiness and agoraphobia. This may be relevant to your back or neck pain, as it can contribute to muscular tension and an experience of difficulty in coping with simple tasks which one might expect to be easy. It also adds to your general stress level.

Can you recognize your posture in your parents?

The way that your parents and other older peers use their bodies in posture and mannerisms is a great influence, usually at a subconscious level.

You may develop similar physical ailments to your parents, low back ache perhaps, because you use your body in a similar way and put stress on similar tissues.

Do you respond to stresses in a similar way to your parents?

You not only copy physical responses from your parents, but emotional ones too. Their differing emotional reactions to stress, or lack of them, affect you also. For example, if your mother tended to bottle things up and get a headache when under pressure, you may react in a similar way. This can appear in childhood or sometime later in life. Often focuses of tension are thought of as family weaknesses, such as a weak chest or a sensitive stomach.

What sort of environment were you brought up in?

Childhood influences such as nutrition, schooling and family relationships can set the patterns of tension, health or unease that you have in your body. These can remain an influence for the rest of your life.

Past Events

These are some of the events in your medical history which may be contributing to your back or neck pain. They may have occurred some time ago, but unless you have recovered from them fully, they can continue to have an effect on your health.

Have you had any major illnesses?

Different illnesses affect individuals in different ways, and the degree of recovery varies. In certain illnesses recovery can take months; sometimes individuals never totally recover and the illness leaves its mark on the person's tissues. For example, hepatitis is a moderately severe illness that most people recover from within about six weeks; some, however, continue to have symptoms of poor liver function, such as intolerance of fatty foods, for years afterwards. The quality of their tissues has changed, and this can contribute to muscular aches and pains. There are many other illnesses that can have subtle long-term effects, notably glandular fever, meningitis, malaria, typhoid and other tropical diseases.

Have you had any operations?

The reasons why you had surgical treatment and the possible functional changes to your body as a result (such as losing your ovaries after a total hysterectomy) are obviously important factors in contributing to your current state. Other points to consider are the effects of scar tissue at the site of the operation, and possible trauma during the operation. For example, the extraction of wisdom teeth can involve pressure on the jaw, which may contribute to jaw, head and neck symptoms. Scars tend to tighten the tissues around them, and may be tender and irritable. An appendix or hernia scar in the lower part of the abdomen can sometimes affect the function of the pelvis on that side and contribute to sacro-iliac problems. Surgery also has major effects on the function of the spine (see Surgery p.117).

Have you had any major accidents?

The influence of these depends on their severity, what was affected and when they occurred. A broken leg in childhood can occasionally affect growth in the limb, causing a limp and uneven pelvic and spinal curves to compensate. A broken leg in an adult, however, is less likely to cause shortening of the limb, and has little effect on the fitness of the spine.

Car crashes and other such accidents are usually underestimated in their potential to cause widespread long-term damage; even in the absence of obvious injury, considerable disruption can occur under the surface (see Trauma p.74). It may be days before the shock begins to wear off and symptoms such as headaches, lethargy, low back pain, confusion and chest pain begin to appear. These events can affect the patterns of tension in your body and contribute to subsequent problems.

Have you had back or neck pain before?

If your problem has been recurring over many years, it suggests that the factors causing it need to be analyzed carefully if permanent relief is to be obtained. If your problem started in your teens (or earlier), it suggests that there is some basic anomaly or postural problem that may be difficult to change. Nonetheless you can usually improve your body's ability to compensate for it and so suffer no symptoms. Major problems in the past, such as a herniated disc, are prone to recurrence.

General Health

How do you feel in yourself? What is your general level of vitality?

In order for you, as a whole, to be healthy, all of your parts have to be functioning well. If the answers to these questions are not good, you need to investigate further to discover the causes of your problem.

Major disturbances in the heart, lungs and circulation can cause severe symptoms: any breathlessness, fainting or dizzy spells, chest pains, swollen ankles and unexplained fatigue should be investigated. Problems in the heart and lungs can cause a lot of tension and pain in the thoracic area, and treatment to improve the function of the chest and thorax can reduce the tension and ease discomfort, encouraging the healing process (see Visceral Problems p.154).

The food that you eat is important to your general health, as is the regularity of meals (see Nutrition p.133). Many pains and cramps in the abdomen are due to the mobility of the stomach, intestines or colon being upset, as they are made of muscle which can get tense or function with poor coordination. This can also cause stasis, wind, indigestion, constipation and diarrhoea. Colon spasms can also be felt as pain in the low back and contribute to tension there.

Maintaining Factors

These are the factors that may be stopping you from getting better. If a problem has been going on for some time, or is recurrent, you shouldn't just ask yourself 'What is wrong?' but also 'Why hasn't it got better?' Treatment should be concerned with identifying and removing these obstacles to health, as the body is good at healing or adapting to most problems, given the opportunity.

Occasionally problems are self-maintaining, as the symptoms themselves cause stress and tension, which perpetuate the problem even though the original triggering factor may have gone.

Is there anything that is worrying you?

It is well known how distressing events such as divorce and bereavement can be, but it is surprising how stressful even 'positive' events can be, such as moving house, getting married or starting a new job. You should also consider subconscious and emotional undercurrents of stress, such as feeling lonely and lacking in confidence, or having problems in a relationship. Many factors, from both within and without, add together to affect you as a whole (see Stress p.143).

Are you involved in any physical activity that might be maintaining this problem?

Sometimes occupational hazards, sports stresses and hobbies can prevent your recovery. Posture is also important in this respect. Sitting in a badly designed seat all day may prevent a disc problem from healing properly, while straining your eyes, arms and neck at a computer terminal may perpetuate your headaches.

Do you need a rest or a holiday?

Back and neck pains are frequently warning signs that you have reached the point where your tissues cannot cope with any further demands; you need a good rest or holiday to give yourself a proper chance to unwind.

Do you look after your body?

Maintaining a level of fitness sufficient to meet the demands that you put on yourself is essential (see General Fitness p.126). Prevention is better than cure, but poor health hampers both.

How are you reacting to your back or neck pain?

Just having a problem can be extremely stressful. This is particularly so with back and neck pain, as it is not immediately visible to other people and its severity can vary from a mild ache to incapacitating pain. Unless other people have had severe pain themselves, they may dismiss it and ask what the fuss is about. Don't let them, or your problem, worry you unduly. The chances are heavily in your favour that it will clear up quickly.

Conclusion

Having read this chapter you should have some understanding of the factors that may have influenced your present state. You may also have realized that back and neck pains are not simple problems with one cause and one solution, but do

A Typical Case of Low Back Ache

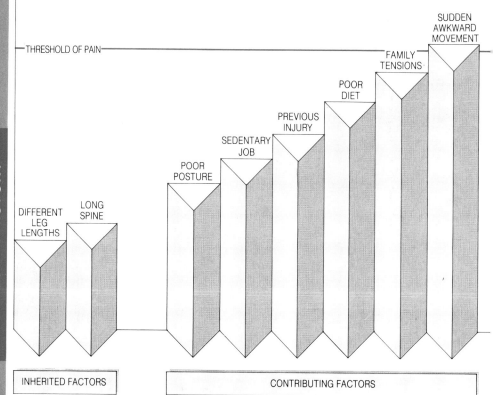

not be disheartened – you can sort them out.

You may also have asked yourself 'What about the actual event that seemed to trigger off this problem?' This may have been important, for example, a major trauma, bad shock or lifting something heavy, or it may have been relatively trivial. Often many factors add together over a long period of time, until only a minor event seems to trigger off a lot of problems. Some problems therefore seem to come on for no apparent reason, so putting too much emphasis on the immediate cause can be misleading.

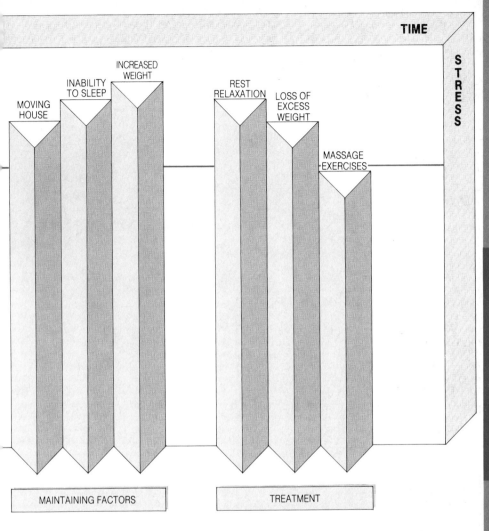

TIME

S
T
R
E
S
S

INCREASED
WEIGHT

INABILITY
TO SLEEP

MOVING
HOUSE

REST
RELAXATION

LOSS OF
EXCESS
WEIGHT

MASSAGE
EXERCISES

MAINTAINING FACTORS

TREATMENT

There is a constant dynamic exchange between the ability of your mind and body to heal, deal with and compensate for the stresses that occur in and around you. As your level of stress increases, your ability to cope with further demands decreases. It is only when the threshold is reached that symptoms occur. Simply relieving the symptoms, therefore, may not be enough if your system is left near this threshold, making the problem, or another one, likely to recur. Good treatment and prevention are then necessary for the levels of stress and tension to decrease.

Diagnose Your Problem

This chapter will analyze your specific problems in detail; here you will find each problem dealt with separately under its own heading. To make an accurate diagnosis it is essential to differentiate between the various causes of back and neck pain and to understand your own individual problems. Using this chapter will therefore be easier if you have already consulted the previous chapters.

Using This Chapter

To help you diagnose your problem, this chapter is divided into three main sections, corresponding to the major areas of the spine. You should first check the illustration on the following page to select the appropriate area for your problem, then consult the relevant diagnostic flow chart to which you are referred.

By using the flow charts you should be able to make an accurate diagnosis of your problem. You can then confirm this by consulting the comprehensive list of symptoms included under each heading. You are then referred to the appropriate self-help methods of treating your problems and preventing it from recurring: these will be found in Chapter Five and Chapter Six. As well as a discussion of the likely causes, each entry gives an idea of the course you can expect your problem to take.

Points to Note Some problems can originate in one area and cause problems in another.

■ If you have symptoms in your low back, buttocks or legs, check all three charts in the Low Back Area section.

■ If you have shoulder problems, check the charts in the Neck Area and the Thoracic Area sections.

■ Muscular tension occurs as part of any problem and is also the cause of most. You should always consult the section dealing with this.

Warning While the problems described in this book cover most causes of back and neck pain, you should consult a qualified therapist if you

■ do not start to get better within two weeks;

■ feel generally ill and feverish;

■ have recurrent abdominal or pelvic pains;

■ suffer from unremitting pain, which is worse at night;

■ have severe pins and needles in your arms or legs;

■ have severe numbness in your arms or legs;

■ are afraid and want reassurance.

DIAGNOSIS

The Areas of the Spine

This chapter is divided into three main sections, which correspond to the major areas of the spine. Each section covers the spine and the related areas of the body where symptoms may also be experienced: in the Low Back Area (p.33) symptoms can be felt in the buttocks, groin and legs; in the Thoracic Area (p.54) symptoms can be felt around the ribs or in the front of the chest; in the Neck Area (p.63) symptoms can be felt in the head, arms or shoulders.

If the symptoms cover more than one area, as is frequently the case with muscular tension, then consult all the relevant sections.

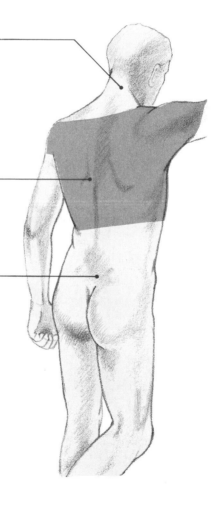

Neck Area
This section includes your neck, throat, head, face and arms. You should consult both the Arm Symptoms chart on p.64 and the Neck Area chart on p.63.

Thoracic Area
This section includes your shoulders, ribs and chest. You should consult the Thoracic Area chart on p.54

Low Back Area
This section includes the area from your lowest ribs via your pelvis to your legs and feet. You should consult all three charts which cover this area:

■ Low Back Area – Recurring Pain (p.33)
■ Low Back Area – Sudden Attack of Pain (p.34)
■ Low Back Area – Hip, Buttock and Leg Symptoms (p.36)

LOW BACK AREA

Low Back Area – Recurring Pain

Persistent pain or ache in the low back area. Lumbago-type back ache.

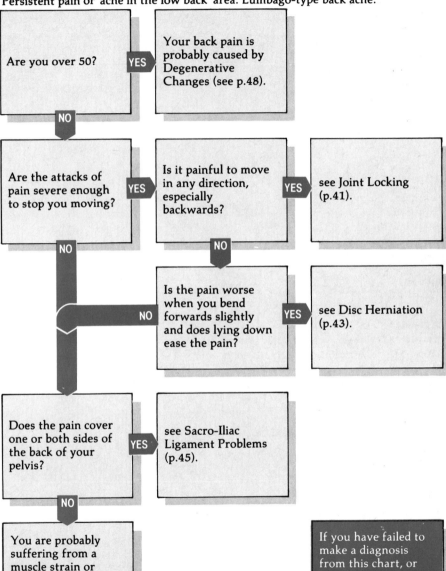

Are you over 50?

YES → Your back pain is probably caused by Degenerative Changes (see p.48).

NO

Are the attacks of pain severe enough to stop you moving?

YES → Is it painful to move in any direction, especially backwards?

YES → see Joint Locking (p.41).

NO →

NO → Is the pain worse when you bend forwards slightly and does lying down ease the pain?

YES → see Disc Herniation (p.43).

NO

Does the pain cover one or both sides of the back of your pelvis?

YES → see Sacro-Iliac Ligament Problems (p.45).

NO

You are probably suffering from a muscle strain or spasm as a result of Muscular Tension (see p.39).

If you have failed to make a diagnosis from this chart, or if your symptoms persist, consult a qualified therapist.

DIAGNOSIS

33

Low Back Area – Sudden Attack of Pain

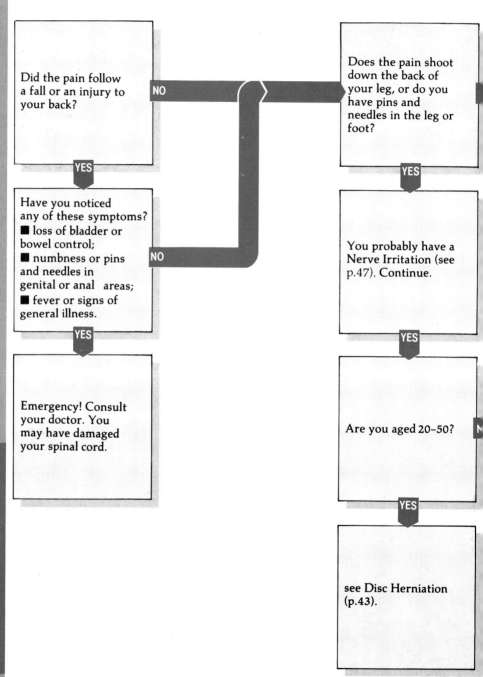

Did the pain follow a fall or an injury to your back?

NO

Does the pain shoot down the back of your leg, or do you have pins and needles in the leg or foot?

YES

Have you noticed any of these symptoms?
■ loss of bladder or bowel control;
■ numbness or pins and needles in genital or anal areas;
■ fever or signs of general illness.

NO

You probably have a Nerve Irritation (see p.47). Continue.

YES

YES

Emergency! Consult your doctor. You may have damaged your spinal cord.

Are you aged 20–50?

YES

see Disc Herniation (p.43).

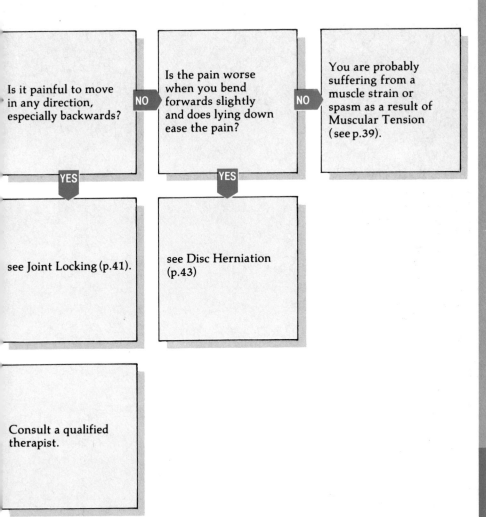

Is it painful to move in any direction, especially backwards? **NO** → Is the pain worse when you bend forwards slightly and does lying down ease the pain? **NO** → You are probably suffering from a muscle strain or spasm as a result of Muscular Tension (see p.39).

YES

see Joint Locking (p.41).

YES

see Disc Herniation (p.43)

Consult a qualified therapist.

If you fail to make a diagnosis from this chart, or if your symptoms persist, consult a qualified therapist.

Low Back Area – Hip, Buttock and Leg Symptoms

Pain, numbness or pins and needles.

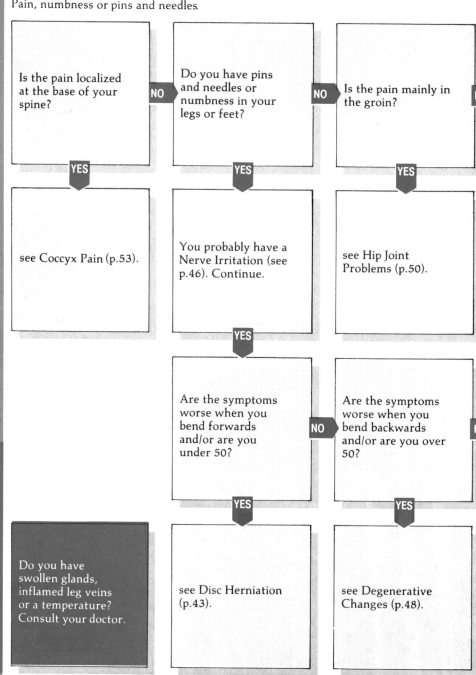

Is the pain localized at the base of your spine?

NO

Do you have pins and needles or numbness in your legs or feet?

NO

Is the pain mainly in the groin?

N

YES

see Coccyx Pain (p.53).

YES

You probably have a Nerve Irritation (see p.46). Continue.

YES

see Hip Joint Problems (p.50).

YES

Are the symptoms worse when you bend forwards and/or are you under 50?

NO

Are the symptoms worse when you bend backwards and/or are you over 50?

N

Do you have swollen glands, inflamed leg veins or a temperature? Consult your doctor.

YES

see Disc Herniation (p.43).

YES

see Degenerative Changes (p.48).

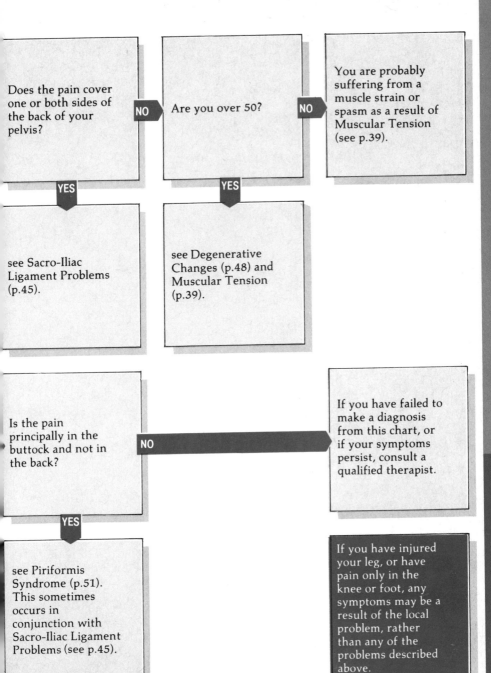

Does the pain cover one or both sides of the back of your pelvis?

NO → Are you over 50?

NO → You are probably suffering from a muscle strain or spasm as a result of Muscular Tension (see p.39).

YES ↓

see Sacro-Iliac Ligament Problems (p.45).

YES ↓

see Degenerative Changes (p.48) and Muscular Tension (p.39).

Is the pain principally in the buttock and not in the back?

NO → If you have failed to make a diagnosis from this chart, or if your symptoms persist, consult a qualified therapist.

YES ↓

see Piriformis Syndrome (p.51). This sometimes occurs in conjunction with Sacro-Iliac Ligament Problems (see p.45).

If you have injured your leg, or have pain only in the knee or foot, any symptoms may be a result of the local problem, rather than any of the problems described above.

Acute Low Back Pain – What to do in an Emergency

■ Don't panic! No matter how severe the pain, panic does not help. Be reassured that no matter how bad it feels, the chances of it being due to any major damage are very small.

■ Lie down – on the floor if you can't get to a bed. The best position is with your knees bent up and your low back flattened against the floor (see Pelvic Tilt (see p.123). You may also find a chair or cushions under your knees more comfortable.

■ Try to relax by taking deep, slow breaths.

■ Take a painkiller if you wish (see Medicines p.116).

■ Follow the flow charts in the Low Back Area section of this chapter to make an initial diagnosis. The three most likely causes in an acute case are:

1 Muscular Tension or spasm (p.39).

2 Joint Locking (p.41).

3 Disc Herniation (p.43).

Treatment
As a general guide the following measures will relieve most cases:

■ Bedrest for 24 to 48 hours (p.88).

■ Relaxation (p.79).

■ Gentle Massage (p.82), if you can stand it.

■ If you have to move support yourself with a stick, a corset or a belt done up tightly low down.

■ As the pain subsides do the Low Back Stretch (p.98) then progress to the complete Mild Routine.

Muscular Tension

Aching in the low back, often called 'lumbago', is mostly caused by the muscles. Tension is a result of muscles contracting tighter than their normal tone and is often associated with tension in other areas. If it is maintained for a long time the muscles may become stringy or 'fibrotic'. Extreme contraction or cramp is called 'spasm'.

Symptoms

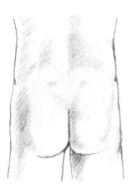

■ Aching over the tense muscles. As several muscles are usually affected, the ache may be vague and cover a wide area, including both sides of your back, your buttocks and legs. These locations may vary with changing circumstances. Spasm may be more severely painful and more localized.

■ The ache may vary in intensity and duration. It can seem to go then return hours, days or weeks later.

■ The muscles feel hard, bunched up and tender to pressure.

■ The area where the muscles are tight may feel stiff when you move. This may ease with further movements as the muscles warm up. Due to this the muscles can feel particularly stiff first thing in the morning, then ease after a few minutes.

■ The muscles may contract so strongly that they pull you into an awkward or crooked posture.

■ Stretching the tight muscle produces a pulling sensation, but there is some elasticity, so that you may be able to ease the tightness by stretching further.

■ The tension is eased if you are lying down or supporting your back.

■ Simple muscular tension does not involve any nerve symptoms such as pins and needles or numbness in a leg or foot.

Causes

Many factors add together to produce muscular tension. These include poor posture, exhaustion, weak abdominal muscles, overweight, emotional upsets and worries, cold temperatures and problems in related tissues.

Muscular spasm may occur as a protective reflex when a structure is damaged or diseased, for example, a herniated disc.

Treatment
- Rest (p.78).

- Relaxation (p.79).

- Heat (p.90).

- Massage (p.82).

- Painkillers can help if the pain is more severe, (see Medicines p.116).

- Low Back Stretch (p.98); progress to the complete Mild Routine.

Leg Pain

The most frequently occurring pattern of muscular tension associated with low back pain is tension in the buttock and down the outside or back of the thigh to the knee. This is usually on one side only, although it may occur on both. This muscular tension is often called 'sciatica' in the mistaken belief that it is caused by irritation of the sciatic nerve. Treatment is as for muscular tension, and the leg responds particularly well to the massage of the painful muscles themselves. Prognosis is good. If it recurs it may be partly caused by a short leg on the opposite side (see Side To Side Posture p.123).

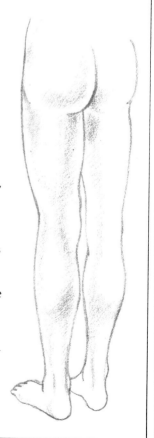

Prevention Most of the sections in Chapter Five – Prevent Your Problem Recurring and Chapter Six – Risk Factors to Avoid will help prevent muscular tension. You should consult in particular:

■ Posture (p.121).

■ Regular Exercise (p.127).

■ Lifting (p.130)

■ Excess Weight (p.139).

■ Occupational Hazards (p.140).

Prognosis Good for immediate relief using the treatments outlined above. Understanding the reasons why your muscles are tense is important to prevent future recurrences. You should read Chapter One – How Your Spine Works and Chapter Two – Take Your Personal Case History.

Joint Locking

The exact process that occurs when a joint locks is debatable, but it is thought most likely to be a spasm of the small muscles immediately surrounding the joint.

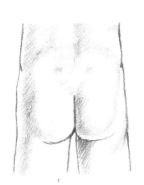

Symptoms ■ This usually occurs suddenly without any warning or build-up although you may have had muscular tension in the area.

■ The joint may have locked while you were not in an upright position – for example, when you were bending forwards – in which case you may be stuck in that position. Alternatively, you may be able to stand, but only in a crooked way.

■ You cannot move the locked joint in any direction: it is painful even to try to do so. If you stay still the pain is much reduced.

■ The pain is worst when you try to bend backwards and towards the side of the worst pain.

■ The pain is localized to the joint affected and is usually felt more on one side. Occasionally there may be pain in the leg.

■ There are no nerve symptoms, such as pins and needles or numbness in the feet or legs.

Causes The locking is a problem of function rather than disease. It can happen to anyone and is usually the result of a quick or unguarded movement, particularly twisting. Individuals with loose joints and tense muscles are more susceptible.

Treatment ■ Don't panic! This will increase the pain.

■ If the pain is very severe get into as comfortable a position as possible, supporting yourself with cushions if necessary, and don't move until it eases slightly.

■ Rest (p.78).

■ Relaxation (p.79).

■ Heat (p.90).

■ Massage (p.82).

■ If the pain is severe you might consider using muscle relaxants (see Medicines p.116).

■ Support (p.89).

■ Low Back Stretch (p.98). Progress to the complete Mild Routine.

Prevention Most of the sections in Chapter Five – Prevent Your Problem From Recurring and Chapter Six – Risk Factors to Avoid will help prevent underlying muscular tension. You should particularly consult the following:

■ Posture (p.121).

■ Regular Exercise (p.127).

■ Excess Weight (p.139).

■ Occupational Hazards (p.140).

Prognosis Good. Most cases of locked joints gradually ease by themselves within a few days. The exercises will then help you to get the joint fully mobile. Occasionally either it doesn't resolve itself or you may need quicker relief, in which case you should consult a qualified therapist. In straightforward cases the therapist manipulates the joint, so that it clicks and releases the muscle spasm, giving instant relief, although the therapist you consult may relieve the pain by other methods.

Disc Herniation

Most low back problems that are called 'slipped discs' are not due to discs at all – they are incorrectly diagnosed. True disc problems are relatively rare, but when they do occur they can be severe and need special care. Over ninety-five per cent of disc problems occur at the very base of the back, where the lowest two discs can bulge or herniate.

Symptoms

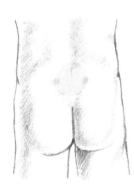

■ Pain in the low back, centrally and to one or both sides.

■ The pain may spread into the buttocks and down one, or rarely, both legs.

■ Sitting and standing are painful, but lying down gives relief.

■ The pain is characteristically worse first thing in the morning, as the disc swells overnight while there is no weight on it.

■ Coughing, sneezing, or any jarring movements may hurt.

■ Nerve symptoms, such as numbness or pins and needles in a leg or foot, may be present. If you are between the ages of twenty and fifty these are most likely to be caused by disc problems, so their presence is a good diagnostic indicator.

■ You may find yourself standing crookedly, as your muscles are in spasm to protect the disc from further damage.

■ Bending forwards is particularly painful and you may only be able to go a few degrees. It is usually worse if you combine it with bending away from the side of worst pain. Either of these two movements may also aggravate the nerve symptoms.

■ Bending backwards is often not as painful as it would be in Joint Locking (p.41).

Causes

Discs are strong structures, so damage to them only tends to occur after an accumulation of minute injuries over many years. For this reason disc problems are rare under the age of twenty.

The disc hardens as you get older, so acute herniation or bulging is rare in people over fifty.

The discs themselves are insensitive to pain, so symptoms only occur when they stretch or irritate other structures. Symptoms can therefore come on rapidly once the 'final straw' has been added. This need not be a major injury: it can be bending forwards, lifting awkwardly or something as simple as a sneeze.

A variety of factors can contribute to the long-term strain on your disc, such as excess weight, poor strength in your stomach muscles or poor flexibility further up your spine. Poor posture and incorrect lifting, if done frequently, can also adversely affect the strength of your discs.

Treatment
- Bedrest (p.88).
- Rest (p.78).
- Relaxation (p.79).
- Traction (p.92).
- Support (p.89).
- Once the symptoms have started to ease, do the Mild Routine (p.96).

Prevention You must avoid straining your low back for many months after the symptoms have eased. You should consider in particular:
- Sitting Posture (p.125).
- Regular Exercise (p.127).
- Lifting (p.130).
- Sleeping (p.132).
- Excess Weight (p.139).

Prognosis If you follow the measures listed above, your disc should be free of symptoms within a month, although it takes approximately eighteen months to regain its original strength, so you have to be patient.

In a few cases the disc doesn't seem to heal. Either a part of the disc is left in the spinal canal and the nerves remain affected, or the disc presses on too many nerves, causing loss of bladder control and paralysis. In both cases surgery may be necessary (see p.119). It is often worth having a second opinion before having an operation. It is also worth noting that a true disc problem cannot be cured by forceful manipulation, no matter who does it, so do not expect any miracles.

Sacro-Iliac Ligament Problems

Women are most susceptible to overstretching and inflammation of these ligaments, especially during and after pregnancy. Men can suffer from this problem too, however. In this condition the joint is usually too loose, rather than too stiff.

Symptoms

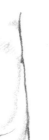

■ Pain or aching over one or both sacro-iliac joints; the tissues over the joints are likely to be tender.

■ The pain may also be felt in the buttock, groin or thigh.

■ The onset of the pain is usually gradual, often for no apparent reason.

■ The pain is worse in movements that might stretch the ligaments, such as turning in bed or getting up from a seat. Repetitive movements or overuse may also aggravate the symptoms, although the effects are occasionally not felt until sometime afterwards.

■ Lying down does not necessarily relieve the pain. You may be comfortable for a while, then the pain will build up again, so that you have to move, and it may wake you at night.

■ Although some movements may be painful, the overall range of them is usually good. You can bend forwards as far as normal, which you would not be able to do if you were suffering from Disc Herniation (p.43) or Joint Locking (p.41).

■ When the ligaments are overstretched the sacro-iliac joints often move too much, so that you might occasionally feel a 'clunk' as the joint shifts from one position to another.

■ There are no nerve symptoms, such as pins and needles or numbness in feet or legs.

Causes   The hormonal changes in pregnancy make the ligaments softer and more vulnerable. This combined with the weight of the baby and uterus means that pregnancy can be a major factor.

Trauma, such as a bad fall, can overstretch the ligaments, but pain is more likely to build up gradually with overuse. Sometimes taking up a new sport, such as golf, or any activity which strains the pelvis, can start it.

Unequal leg lengths or limping can cause the pelvis to be twisted while you are standing and walking, thus putting strain on the ligaments.

Poor flexibility further up the spine, due to factors such as Osteochondritis (p.147), means that more demand is put on the sacro-iliac joint when you move.

Treatment   ■ Ice (p.91).

■ Support (p.89).

■ Massage (p.82).

■ Anti-inflammatory drugs (see Medicines p.116).

■ Avoid any movements that make the pain worse, such as twisting and vigorous exercise.

Prevention   ■ Do the Mild Routine (p.96), concentrating on the Curl-Up and the Cross Arm-Leg Push.

■ See if you have a difference in the length of your legs, (see Side to Side Posture p.123).

■ If the problems is due to repetitive activity, such as an aerobics class or faulty golf swing, either learn to do the activity without straining the joint or give it up.

Prognosis   With care and attention to the causes the inflammation in the overstretched ligaments should calm down in a few days and the pain subside. This is similar to a sprained ankle. Unfortunately it is difficult not to use your sacro-iliac joints, so it can become chronic and persist for many months, in which case you are advised to consult a qualified therapist.

Nerve Irritation

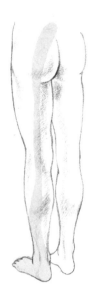

There are a few misconceptions about nerve problems that this section will clear up. You should note that:

■ True nerve problems are uncommon.

■ Nerves do not generally get trapped; they usually suffer from an irritation caused by another structure in the spine.

■ Pain is not a major feature of nerve irritation and many cases occur without it. If it does occur it is a deep 'burning' pain going down to the foot or sometimes an intermittent 'shooting' pain.

In the absence of pins and needles or numbness in the legs, leg pain should not be ascribed to nerves. If you assume that leg pain is due to nerves, you may not carry out the necessary treatment. Most pain in the legs is caused by Muscular Tension (p.39).

Symptoms ■ The most common symptoms are pins and needles or numbness in the leg or foot.

■ Less commonly there may be weakness of the muscles in the leg, especially the calf, or shrinkage of the muscles in the leg.

■ If the nerve is irritated by a disc herniation, the pain will be worse if you bend forwards. This is the most likely cause for people between the ages of twenty and fifty.

Straight Leg Raising Test

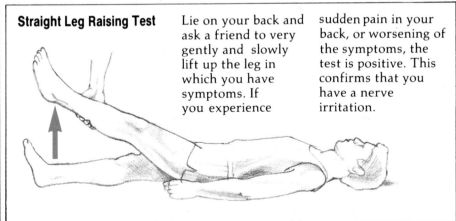

Lie on your back and ask a friend to very gently and slowly lift up the leg in which you have symptoms. If you experience sudden pain in your back, or worsening of the symptoms, the test is positive. This confirms that you have a nerve irritation.

■ If the nerve is irritated by degenerative changes in the disc, bone or joints, the nerve symptoms will be worse when you bend backwards and towards the side of the problem. This is most likely over the age of fifty.

Causes

■ Disc Herniation (p.43).

■ Degenerative Changes (p.48).

■ Piriformis Syndrome (p.51).

There are many other less common causes of nerve symptoms, some of them potentially serious. You should consult a specialist if you

■ have pins and needles in the front of your thigh, or in your buttock or groin;

■ have persistent or worsening symptoms;

■ have pins and needles or numbness in both legs;

■ lose control of your bladder or bowel functions.

Treatment and Prognosis

The treatment depends on the cause, so you should refer to the appropriate sections. The nerves usually recover once the irritation is removed.

Degenerative Changes

These are natural changes that occur in everybody with age, caused by wear and tear. In some people, however, they occur more extensively than in others. The changes involve the discs and vertebral bodies (see Aging p.149) and the joints, from osteoarthritis (see Arthritis p.146).

Usually the degenerative changes themselves give no symptoms; many people of advanced age with obvious degenerative changes in their spines have no pain. The changes may contribute, however, to muscular tension, and it is usually the muscles that give the pain in these cases. Unfortunately any aches and pains are usually ascribed to the degenerative changes rather than to the muscles, so no treatment is given and people are incorrectly told that they have to live with the pain rather than obtaining relief.

DIAGNOSIS

X-rays are an accurate, if limited, way of assessing the state of the bones, but note that the degree of change seen on X-rays bears little relation to the severity of the symptoms.

Symptoms

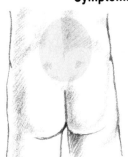

■ Stiffness and a reduction in the range of the movements allowed by the back.

■ Occasionally the joint degeneration causes a deep ache which can be worse when the back is kept stationary. This occurs when the osteoarthritis is in an active inflammatory phase.

■ Occasionally the changes may result in a nerve irritation, causing symptoms such as tingling or numbness in a foot or leg. In such cases you should consult a qualified therapist.

Causes

Degenerative changes begin as early as your twenties, but the effects are not usually noticed until your fifties or later. The greater the strain on your back the more the degenerative changes, thus the process may be accelerated by excess weight, incorrect lifting, trauma to the back from sports stresses, bad posture, osteochondritis and certain occupational hazards.

Treatment

Inflammation in an active phase of osteoarthritis can be treated with the following:

■ Anti-inflammatory drugs (see Medicines p.116).

■ Rest (p.78).

There is no treatment for the degenerative changes themselves, but muscular tension can be treated by the following:

■ Relaxation (p.79).

■ Heat (p.90).

■ Massage (p.82).

■ Mild Routine (p.96).

Prevention

Keep your spine mobile as you get older by attention to the following:

■ Posture (p.121).

■ Regular Exercise (p.127).

■ Warmth (p.137).

Although the degenerative changes are not reversible, many elderly people, with considerable degenerative changes in their spines, have no discomfort whatsoever. In theory, therefore, most people should be able to be relieved of their discomfort with the proper treatment and attention to muscular tension.

Hip Joint Problems

Full consideration of all the problems that can arise in the hip joint is outside the scope of this book.

The hip joint in adults is a strong joint and is only affected with any frequency by arthritis. Hip problems are unlikely to occur under fifty years of age. Hip pain and limping in children should be looked at by a doctor or specialist as soon as possible.

Symptoms

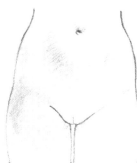

■ Pain is felt in the groin, inside the thigh and in the buttock. It may also be referred to the knee. Pain on the outside of the buttock and thigh (often called the hip) is usually due to muscular tension.

■ The pain is usually a nagging ache and may occur at any time – sometimes even at night.

■ One or both hips can be affected.

■ Stiffness occurs progressively as the wear and tear advances. In severe cases you may limp and walking can be difficult.

Hip Test

Lie on your back, bend your knee up to ninety degrees, then twist it either way. If you feel pain in your groin it is likely to be caused by your hip joint. The worst affected hip is less mobile than the other one.

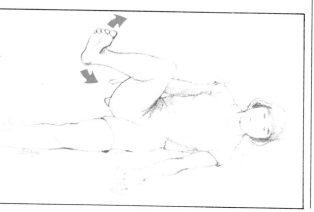

Causes Wear and tear with age (see Arthritis p.146). Some individuals are more prone to this than others. If you are overweight throughout your life or are on your feet all day then the hip joints take more strain.

Treatment There is no treatment to reverse osteoarthritic changes. In many cases, however, there is tension in the deep muscles around the joint that can be eased by the following:

■ Heat (p.90).

■ Massage (p.82).

■ Leg Swinging Exercise (p.94).

■ If the pain in the hip is severe, anti-inflammatory drugs (see Medicines p.116). Ask your doctor for advice.

Prevention You should aim to keep your hip joint as mobile as possible throughout your life by attention to the following:

■ Regular Exercise (p.127).

■ Posture (p.121).

■ Excess Weight (p.139).

■ Occupational Hazards (p.140).

Prognosis In mild cases the treatments outlined above can ease the symptoms and you may have no severe problems. Some cases, however, do advance so that the joint becomes very arthritic, in which case surgical hip replacement is the only solution. This is one of the most successful orthopaedic operations, giving great relief in most cases.

Piriformis Syndrome

This is tension or spasm in one of the deep muscles in the buttock, called the piriformis, which runs from the sacrum to the top of the thigh. It is important because in a percentage of people the sciatic nerve passes through the muscle, so tightness in the muscle can irritate the nerve and cause symptoms, such as pins and needles or numbness in a foot or leg.

Symptoms
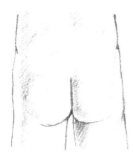

■ Pain deep in the centre of the buttock, which may spread down the back of the thigh, especially if the hamstrings are also tight.

■ Vague tingling in the lower leg and foot. This is not as defined as a Nerve Irritation (p.47).

■ The muscle is tender to touch and feels hard and lumpy.

■ Movements of the lower spine are free and give no symptoms or pain.

■ This syndrome can also be associated with Sacro-Iliac Ligament Problems (p.45) and Hip Joint Problems (p.50).

■ The pain in the buttock tends to be worse when you sit for a long time, or when standing on the leg and twisting, such as when playing golf.

Causes This is usually the result of a build up of tension from a number of factors such as emotional or sexual tension, poor posture and stress. Some people stand with their buttocks clenched which can contribute to the problem.

Treatment ■ Massage (p.82).

■ Relaxation (p.79).

■ Leg Swinging Exercise (p.94)

Prevention ■ Regular Exercise (p.127).

■ Posture (p.121).

■ Stress (p.143).

Prognosis Good. The pain usually disappears within a few days or weeks.

Piriformis Test

You can test to see if the muscle is tight by standing on the affected leg and twisting your body around it, so that your foot points inwards. The test is positive if it causes pain in the buttock or pins and needles in the leg or foot.

Coccyx Pain

The coccyx is made up of four small bones joined by ligaments to the lower tip of the sacrum. It is the non-functioning remains of a tail.

Symptoms

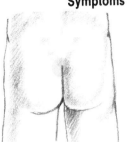

■ The pain is localized to the tip of the sacrum over the coccyx. It is usually tender to touch.

■ Sitting makes the symptoms worse – particularly on a hard surface.

■ There are no nerve symptoms, such as pins and needles or numbness in a leg or foot.

■ Movements of the low back are unrestricted and painless.

Causes

A fall on to the base of the spine or, rarely, direct trauma from a blow to the coccyx. In some cases the coccyx may be fractured, although usually it is the ligaments between the sacrum and the coccyx that are pulled.

Some cases that come on without an obvious injury can be due to tension in the small muscle either side of the coccyx, called the coccygeus. This may be aggravated by habitual tensing of the buttocks or anxieties about the pelvic area. It can also be associated with problems such as piles or constipation. In women scarring of the pelvic floor following a difficult labour can cause the area to tighten up.

Treatment

■ Avoid irritating the coccyx further by sitting on a soft surface or with a cushion under both buttocks so that there is no direct pressure on the centre. In very sensitive cases sitting on an inflatable ring may be more comfortable.

■ Massage (p.82).

Prevention

Falls and blows are hard to prevent. Tension in the area can be avoided by the following:

■ Regular Exercise (p.127).

■ Breathing Pattern (p.135).

Prognosis

This depends on severity. Usually it settles down within a few weeks.

Thoracic Area

Pain or stiffness in your mid-back

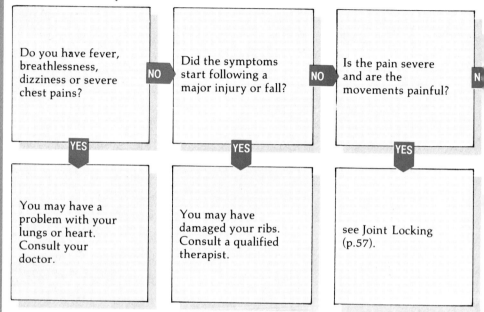

Do you have fever, breathlessness, dizziness or severe chest pains?

NO

Did the symptoms start following a major injury or fall?

NO

Is the pain severe and are the movements painful?

N

YES

YES

YES

You may have a problem with your lungs or heart. Consult your doctor.

You may have damaged your ribs. Consult a qualified therapist.

see Joint Locking (p.57).

If you fail to make a diagnosis from this chart or if your symptoms persist, consult a qualified therapist.

If you have pain in the shoulder see Shoulder Problems (p.59).

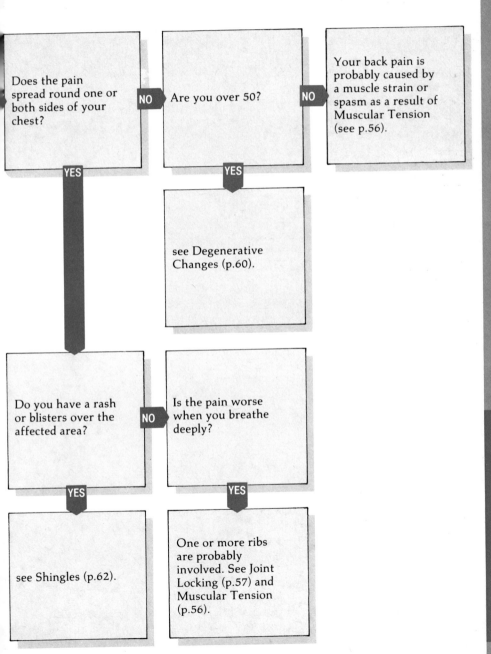

Does the pain spread round one or both sides of your chest?

NO

Are you over 50?

NO

Your back pain is probably caused by a muscle strain or spasm as a result of Muscular Tension (see p.56).

YES

YES

see Degenerative Changes (p.60).

Do you have a rash or blisters over the affected area?

NO

Is the pain worse when you breathe deeply?

YES

YES

see Shingles (p.62).

One or more ribs are probably involved. See Joint Locking (p.57) and Muscular Tension (p.56).

Muscular Tension

Pain in the thoracic area is usually muscular in origin. Tension is a result of the muscles contracting tighter than their normal tone and is often associated with tension in other areas. If it is maintained for a long time the muscles become stringy or 'fibrotic'. Extreme contraction or cramp is called 'spasm'.

Symptoms

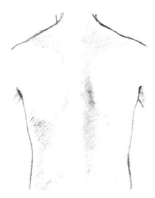

■ Aching in the muscles that are tense, which may be in the back, between your shoulders, round your ribs on either side, or even in the front of your chest.

■ The ache will be worse the more you contract the muscles or use them to work, thus it tends to build up as the day goes on. They may also feel stiff first thing in the morning.

■ The muscles are hard and tender to pressure. They may feel stringy if they have been contracted for a long time.

■ If the tension becomes spasm, you may feel severe pain, which can double you up or cause you to bend to one side.

■ Stretching the muscles gives a tight, pulling sensation.

■ Breathing deeply may be uncomfortable and some of your upper body movements may feel stiff and restricted.

Causes Muscular tension in the thoracic area affects most people from time to time. Muscles do not like continuous static use, but they can keep up intermittent use, such as normal movement, all day. Sometimes, however, tension can build up and become quite severe. It is usually the result of a combination of factors: stooping posture, especially in tall or round-shouldered people; overwork; emotional worries, which can cause tension across the shoulders; poor breathing pattern and lung problems, such as asthma and bronchitis; cold temperatures; jobs where muscles are used continuously, such as typing or bending over a desk; lack of exercise, so that the muscles are never stretched.

Treatment	■ Rest (p.78).
	■ Relaxation (p.79).
	■ Heat (p.90).
	■ Massage (p.82).
	■ Sitting Routine (p.112).

Prevention	Most of the sections in Chapter Five – Prevent Your Problem Recurring and Chapter Six – Risk Factors to Avoid will help prevent muscular tension. You should consult in particular:
	■ Posture (p.121).
	■ Regular Exercise (p.127).
	■ Breathing (p.135).
	■ Occupational Hazards (p.140).

Prognosis	Good for immediate relief. Long-term prevention depends on you using this book to understand the causes of the problem and what you can do about them.

Joint Locking

There are two sets of joints involved in this area

1 The intervertebral joints.

2 The joints between the vertebrae and the ribs.

The mechanism of joint locking is a matter of controversy, but it appears to be a spasm of the small muscles immediately surrounding a joint. In the case of a rib this can cause the rib to be held in an awkward position, such as in a breathing-in position when the other ribs are breathing out. In general, however, this is not as dramatic as joint locking in either the neck area or the low back area as the thoracic area moves much less.

Symptoms 1	■ Pain over, or just to the side of, a particular vertebra or small group of vertebrae.
	■ The muscles around the locked joint feel hard and tender to touch.
	■ Movement in any direction is painful.

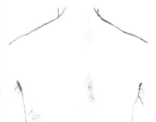

■ If an upper thoracic vertebra is involved, movements of the neck may feel restricted and painful.

■ The pain occasionally spreads into the shoulders and upper arms.

■ Joint locking does not cause any nerve symptoms, such as pins and needles.

Symptoms 2

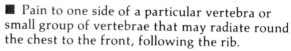

■ Pain to one side of a particular vertebra or small group of vertebrae that may radiate round the chest to the front, following the rib.

■ The muscles around the locked rib feel hard and tender to touch.

■ Movement in any direction is painful.

■ Deep breathing may also be painful.

■ The pain occasionally spreads into the shoulders and upper arms.

■ Joint locking does not cause any nerve symptoms, such as pins and needles.

Causes

In this area it is usually due to a chronic build-up of muscular tension. It is more likely to occur if your muscles are already tense, but can happen to anybody. It can also occur suddenly, as a result of an awkward twisting movement or cough.

Treatment

■ Don't panic! This will increase the pain.

■ If the pain is severe get into as comfortable a position as possible, supporting yourself with cushions if necessary; don't move until it eases.

■ Heat (p.90).

■ Massage (p.82).

■ Support (p.89).

■ If the pain is severe you might consider using painkillers or muscle relaxants (see Medicines p.116).

Prevention

It is very difficult to guard against joint locking, however, you can reduce the risks by considering the following:

■ Regular Exercise (p.127).

DIAGNOSIS

- Breathing (p.135).

- Occupational Hazards (p.140).

Prognosis Good. Most cases of locked joints ease by themselves in two or three days. In some cases the acute pain subsides but the joint or rib remains in an awkward position. This can become a chronic problem, niggling in the background and flaring up in times of stress. It is best to get this moving either by exercise, especially swimming, or by having treatment from a qualified therapist.

Shoulder Problems

Symptoms in the shoulder itself can be divided into two categories:

- Muscular tension spreading from the neck or thoracic areas.

- Problems in the shoulder joint itself or the small joint on the point of the shoulder between the collar bone and the shoulder blade (acromio-clavicular joint).

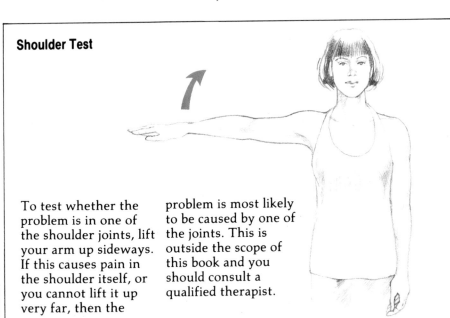

Shoulder Test

To test whether the problem is in one of the shoulder joints, lift your arm up sideways. If this causes pain in the shoulder itself, or you cannot lift it up very far, then the problem is most likely to be caused by one of the joints. This is outside the scope of this book and you should consult a qualified therapist.

Treatment Muscular tension in your shoulder will respond to the following:

- Rest (p.78).
- Relaxation (p.79).
- Heat (p.90).
- Massage (p.82).
- Mild Routine (p.96).
- Sitting Routine (p.112).

Prevention Most of the sections in Chapter Five – Prevent Your Problem Recurring and Chapter Six – Risk Factors to Avoid will help to prevent muscular tension. You should consult in particular:

- Posture (p.121).
- Regular Exercise (p.127).
- Occupational Hazards (p.140).
- Sports Stresses (p.142).

Prognosis Good, for immediate relief. Long-term prevention depends on using this book to understand the causes of the problem and what you can do about them.

Degenerative Changes

These occur gradually as you get older – everyone over the age of fifty has natural wear and tear changes in the thoracic spine. Degenerative changes themselves don't usually cause any pain, but they can contribute to the development of other symptoms, which are principally due to muscular tension.

Symptoms ■ A decrease in the mobility of the spine is a natural consequence of these changes. This is because the discs get thinner and the joints stiffer.

■ Your posture may alter as you get older. In the thoracic area there is usually an increase in the forward bending or round-shouldered posture called a kyphosis. This may be further increased if you have areas of osteochondritis

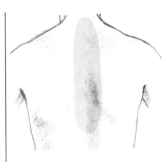

(p.147). The elderly may also be affected by some of the consequences of osteoporosis (see Aging p.149).

■ The mobility of the ribs is slightly affected by advanced degenerative changes, but you can still breathe deeply especially if you use your diaphragm (see Breathing p.135).

■ In the thoracic area the nerves are rarely irritated by degenerative changes, unlike the neck and low back. There should be no pins and needles or numbness in this area.

Causes This is a natural process that occurs with age. It begins in your twenties and carries on for the rest of your life and most people have no ill-effects from it. It is increased in situations where there is an increased strain on the spine over many years from poor posture, excess weight, poor flexibility and old injuries.

Treatment Inflammation in an active phase of osteoarthritis can be treated with the following:

■ Anti-inflammatory drugs (see Medicines p.116).

■ Rest (p.78).

There is no treatment to reverse the natural wear and tear changes that have taken place. However, these are not usually painful and the pain is frequently due to muscular tension, which will respond to the following:

■ Relaxation (p.79).

■ Heat (p.90).

■ Massage (p.82).

■ Mild Routine (p.96).

■ Sitting Routine (p.112).

Prevention Keep your spine mobile as you get older by attention to the following:

■ Regular Exercise (p.127).

■ Posture (p.121).

■ Warmth (p.137).

Prognosis Most elderly people do not suffer pain in the spine due to the natural process of aging, so any discomfort can usually be relieved, using the methods outlined above.

Shingles

This is a nerve infection, caused by the virus that is responsible for chickenpox, called 'herpes zoster', which is not the same as the genital herpes virus. It most frequently affects a nerve in the thoracic area, though it can affect other areas and on rare occasions it can even affect the face.

Symptoms
- This starts with pain along the course of the affected nerve.

- Occurs on one side of the body only, and affects only one or two nerves.

- After two or three days small blisters appear which gradually harden and form scabs.

- After about two weeks the symptoms disappear.

Causes It is thought that the virus lies dormant in the body after childhood chickenpox, and can flare up again if you get exhausted or overstressed. It is more likely to occur in old people.

Treatment There is little that can be done immediately to treat the condition, as the infection has to run its course.

- Rest (p.79) and good Nutrition (p.134) will help your body to fight the virus.

- Do not scratch the blisters, as they may get infected.

- Your doctor may be able to provide you with drugs to ease the symptoms or cold sprays to relieve the pain.

Prognosis Don't be worried that it will spread further, because it won't. The infection usually clears up once it has followed its course. Occasionally the nerve pain can persist for some time after the blisters have gone.

NECK AREA

Neck Area
Pain, stiffness or difficulty moving your neck

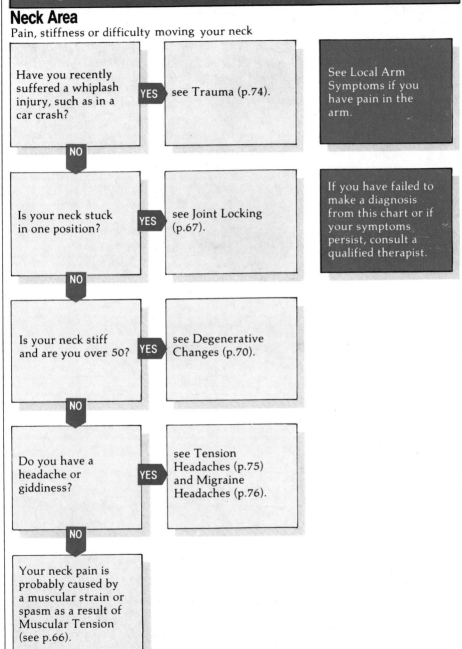

Have you recently suffered a whiplash injury, such as in a car crash? **YES** see Trauma (p.74).

NO

See Local Arm Symptoms if you have pain in the arm.

Is your neck stuck in one position? **YES** see Joint Locking (p.67).

NO

If you have failed to make a diagnosis from this chart or if your symptoms persist, consult a qualified therapist.

Is your neck stiff and are you over 50? **YES** see Degenerative Changes (p.70).

NO

Do you have a headache or giddiness? **YES** see Tension Headaches (p.75) and Migraine Headaches (p.76).

NO

Your neck pain is probably caused by a muscular strain or spasm as a result of Muscular Tension (see p.66).

Arm Symptoms

Pain, numbness or tingling in the arm.

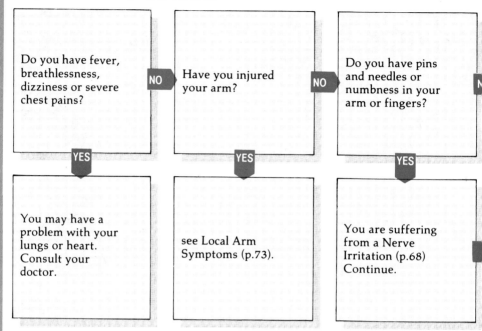

Do you have fever, breathlessness, dizziness or severe chest pains?

NO ▶

Have you injured your arm?

NO ▶

Do you have pins and needles or numbness in your arm or fingers?

N

YES ▼

YES ▼

YES ▼

You may have a problem with your lungs or heart. Consult your doctor.

see Local Arm Symptoms (p.73).

You are suffering from a Nerve Irritation (p.68) Continue.

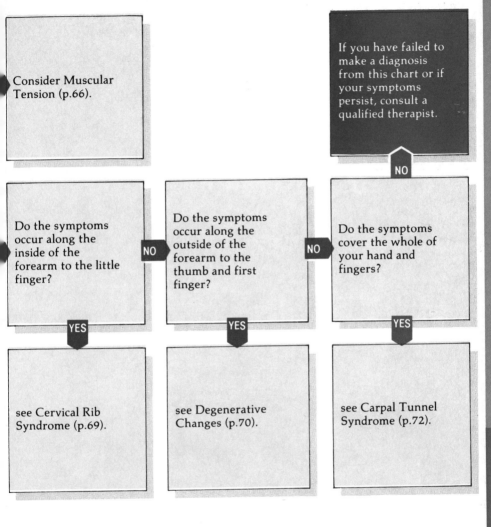

Consider Muscular
Tension (p.66).

If you have failed to
make a diagnosis
from this chart or if
your symptoms
persist, consult a
qualified therapist.

NO

Do the symptoms
occur along the
inside of the
forearm to the little
finger?

NO

Do the symptoms
occur along the
outside of the
forearm to the
thumb and first
finger?

NO

Do the symptoms
cover the whole of
your hand and
fingers?

YES

YES

YES

see Cervical Rib
Syndrome (p.69).

see Degenerative
Changes (p.70).

see Carpal Tunnel
Syndrome (p.72).

DIAGNOSIS

Muscular Tension

This is increased tone in a few or many neck muscles that can vary from mild tightness to severe spasm. It is often associated with tension in other areas. If it is maintained for a long time the muscles may become stringy or 'fibrotic'.

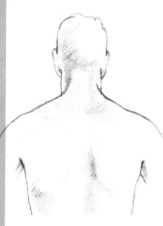

Symptoms

■ Pain or aching in the tense muscles. The ache may be vague, come and go, be on one or both sides and cover a small or wide area. Muscles in the front and sides of the neck may be involved as well as those in the back of the neck.

■ The tension frequently spreads into one or both shoulders.

■ The muscles feel hard and tender to touch.

■ Stiffness in the neck. At the end of a restricted range of movement the muscles are painful to stretch, but there is some elasticity and spring. You may find that the tension eases with gentle stretching.

■ If the upper neck is involved you may also have a Tension Headache (p.75). A severe spasm may even cause dizziness.

■ There are no nerve symptoms, such as pins and needles or numbness in an arm or hand.

Causes

Muscular tension is usually the result of a combination of several factors. There is often a level of background tension which goes unnoticed, until your pain threshold is reached. Factors that may contribute are posture, stress, occupational hazards and trauma.

Treatment

■ Rest (p.78).

■ Relaxation (p.79).

■ Heat (p.90).

■ Massage (p.82).

■ Sitting Routine (p.112).

Prevention

Most of the sections in Chapter Five – Prevent Your Problem Recurring and Chapter Six – Risk Factors to Avoid will help prevent muscular

DIAGNOSIS

tension. You should consult in particular:

- Posture (p.121).
- Regular Exercise (p.127).
- Occupational Hazards (p.140).
- Stress (p.143).

Prognosis Good, for immediate relief. You need to understand the causes in the long-term, otherwise you will be prone to a recurrence of the same problem. Read Chapter Two – Take Your Personal Case History.

Joint Locking

This is thought to be the jamming together of the sliding surfaces of a joint due to local muscular spasm. It may occur in any of the joints of the neck, usually only on one side of the pair of joints on each vertebra. Where the symptoms are more widespread, you may have more than one joint affected. It is sometimes associated with locking of joints in the upper thoracic area and ribs.

Symptoms

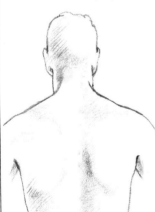

- You cannot turn your neck very far. It may be stuck in an awkward position and you are unable to straighten it.

- Pain over the locked joint. This is usually localized to a small area, although there may be associated muscular tension giving a wider ache.

- The pain can be severe and it can feel as if your whole neck, upper back and shoulders are locked and 'burning'.

- The pain is worst and the movement most limited if you try to turn towards the side of the pain. In severe cases any movement is painful.

- The muscles around the joint are very hard and tender.

- If one of the joints between the top of the neck and the skull is locked you may feel off balance or dizzy and have a headache.

- There are no nerve symptoms, such as pins and needles or numbness in an arm or hand, as a result of a locked joint. Occasionally a deep aching is felt in the arm.

Causes A joint usually locks suddenly as a result of a quick movement, particularly turning the head. This is more likely to happen when you are half awake and your reflexes a little uncoordinated. It sometimes builds up more gradually, for example if your neck is in an awkward position while you are sleeping, or if there is a draught on your neck. It is more likely to happen if there is pre-existing muscular tension or if you have very mobile joints.

Treatment
- Don't panic! This will only increase the pain.
- Rest (p.78).
- Relaxation (p.79).
- Heat (p.90).
- Massage (p.82).
- Support (p.89).
- Do the Head Roll (p.113), then progress to the complete Sitting Routine once the symptoms have eased.
- Neck Lengthening (p.123).

Prevention It is difficult to stop joint locking from occurring. but underlying muscular tension can be reduced by attention to the following:
- Posture (p.121).
- Regular Exercise (p.127).

Prognosis Good. Most cases of joint locking ease within two or three days. Occasionally the acute pain subsides leaving a chronic 'blocked' feeling in your neck, as the joint is still stuck. In such cases you may need to see a qualified therapist who can free the joint.

Nerve Irritation

The nerves in the neck come from the spinal cord and travel out between the vertebrae, over the first rib and down the arm. The symptoms produced by irritation or compression of a nerve are pins and needles, numbness, muscle weakness and sometimes pain. The exact symptoms produced in each case depend on which nerve is affected and where along its course the irritation occurs. The most common sites are:

■ In the spine (neck) itself, caused by Degenerative Changes (p.70) or Trauma (p.74).

■ In the root of the neck over the first rib, as a result of Cervical Rib Syndrome (p.69).

■ In the arm, due to a variety of causes, principally Carpal Tunnel Syndrome (p.72).

Reading the sections on each cause will help you to differentiate between them. The following may act as a rough diagnostic guide.

■ In neck problems due to degenerative changes, the higher nerve roots are usually affected giving symptoms on the outside of the arm to the thumb.

■ In cervical rib syndrome the lower nerve roots are affected, giving symptoms down the inside of the arm to the little finger.

■ In carpal tunnel syndrome the symptoms are felt in the palm of the hand and fingers.

There are many other less common causes of nerve symptoms and full examination can only be done by a specialist: if in doubt consult a qualified therapist.

Cervical Rib Syndrome

(Also known as 'outlet' syndrome.) This is classically due to the development of an extra, or cervical, rib at the base of the neck, which may irritate the nerves as they travel from the spinal cord over the first rib and down the arm. This may also be caused by elevation of the first rib due to muscular tension.

Symptoms ■ Pain or discomfort to one side of the base of the neck, spreading into the upper back and shoulder. In some cases the pain may be severe.

■ Pins and needles, numbness or pain down the inside of the arm to the little finger. There may also be weakness and wasting of some of the small muscles in the hand.

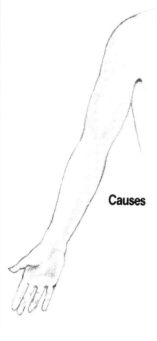

■ The symptoms may be aggravated by carrying heavy shopping bags or stretching the arm. In some cases they arise after sleeping with the arm in an awkward position at night, though care should be taken to distinguish this from Carpal Tunnel Syndrome (p.72).

■ The hollow at the base of the neck behind the collar bone may appear to be filled in; this can give the appearance of having sloping shoulders.

■ X-ray examination may show an extra rib; a fibrous band may not show up on the X-ray.

Causes A true cervical rib or fibrous band is a congenital or developmental problem, so it will have been present all your life; other factors must therefore be contributing to your pain. Postural stresses, such as round shoulders, can contribute, as can fatigue in the muscles and letting your arms hang by your sides, particularly if you are carrying heavy loads. Persistent elevation of the first rib by poor breathing patterns, anxiety and tension, can also contribute. Some individuals have a habit of subconsciously lifting one shoulder when they are worried or under pressure.

Treatment ■ Relaxation (p.79).

■ Sitting Routine (p.112).

■ Massage (p.82).

Prevention ■ Posture (p.121).

■ Breathing (p.135).

Prognosis With consistent care by yourself and, if necessary, a therapist you should be able to relieve most cases of this syndrome. You may need to keep up preventative measures to stop it recurring. In very rare cases surgery may be necessary.

Degenerative Changes

These are natural wear and tear changes that occur in your body as you get older. The principal change in the neck is thinning of the discs, with the formation of small growths of bone, called osteophytes, in some cases. It occurs in the lower half of the neck more extensively than in the upper half. X-ray

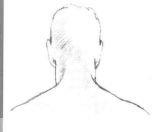

examinations can show the degree of changes, although this often bears little relation to the severity of symptoms.

Symptoms

■ Reduction in the mobility of the neck. The movements become stiffer and their range smaller.

■ Aching may occur in the joints, though this is not always the case; muscles get tight and cause pain.

■ If a nerve is compressed or irritated you may have pins and needles, numbness and pain in one, or sometimes both, arms, particularly on the outside of the arm to the thumb.

■ These nerve symptoms are likely to be worse when you turn and bend your head towards the side of the symptoms, or bend it backwards. This helps to distinguish them from other causes of nerve irritation.

■ In a small percentage of people the degenerative changes cause irritation or compression of the spinal cord. This leads to numbness or pins and needles in the legs as well as the arms; such cases should be under the supervision of a specialist.

Causes

These changes are caused by age; symptoms are therefore unlikely under fifty years of age. In some individuals the process is accelerated, particularly if there has been a previous injury to the neck. Lack of exercise, letting the neck and upper thoracic area get stiff and occupational hazards can also contribute.

Treatment

It is not possible to reverse the degenerative changes once they have occurred; pain caused by muscular tension, however, will respond to the following:

■ Rest (p.78).

■ Relaxation (p.79).

■ Heat (p.90).

■ Massage (p.82).

■ If you are suffering from a nerve irritation, you may need to support your neck (see p.90).

Prevention

Keep your spine mobile as you get older by attention to the following:

■ Posture (p.121).

Regular Exercise (p.127).

Do the Mild Routine (p.96) and the Sitting Routine (p.112).

Prognosis Older people should not resign themselves to chronic discomfort as much can be done to ease pain, using the methods outlined above.

Carpal Tunnel Syndrome

This is the result of an irritation of the median nerve in the front of the wrist, where it passes through an area called the carpal tunnel. It should not be confused with other forms of nerve irritation.

Symptoms ■ Pain, pins and needles, numbness or loss of feeling in the palm of the hand. This is felt particularly in the half of the hand around the thumb and first two or three fingers.

■ Often occurs in both hands.

■ Sometimes weakness is noticeable in one of the small thumb muscles, with the effect that you have difficulty in moving the thumb away from the fingers.

■ The symptoms classically are worst at night, and may wake you up. They are often relieved by shaking the wrist.

■ Movements of your neck should not affect it. This distinguishes it from other causes of nerve irritation.

Causes This can occur for no obvious reason, but it is more likely if you use your hands a lot, as when knitting, in pregnancy, when you have fluid retention, or in conditions such as rheumatoid arthritis.

Treatment ■ Shaking your hand often restores movement to the wrist.

Prevention ■ Stop doing any of the actions that you know bring it on.

■ If you have fluid retention you should reduce your intake of salt.

■ Supplements of B vitamins (especially B6) may help.

Prognosis Variable. It can resolve spontaneously but often needs treatment. If it occurs during pregnancy, it will very likely disappear once you have given birth. If the symptoms steadily worsen, you may need to have the pressure in the carpal tunnel eased by a minor operation; see a qualified therapist for advice.

Local Arm Symptoms

These are symptoms arising from structures in the arm: detailed consideration of these is outside the scope of this book.

Symptoms ■ The muscles in the painful area are hard and tender to touch.

■ Using the arm, such as lifting, makes the symptoms worse.

■ Moving the neck should not affect the symptoms.

■ If you have pins and needles or numbness in an arm or hand, you should consult Nerve Irritation (p.68).

Causes The most common causes of local pain are ligament overstretches and muscular tension; in the arm the latter is often due to overuse. An example of muscular tension is 'tennis elbow', where the forearm muscles get so tight that they pull on their insertion into the bone by the elbow causing an inflammatory reaction.

Treatment ■ Rest (p.78).

■ Relaxation (p.79).

■ Massage (p.82).

Prevention Most of the sections in Chapter Five – Prevent Your Problem Recurring and Chapter Six – Risk Factors to Avoid will help to prevent muscular tension. You should consult in particular:

■ Occupational Hazards (p.140).

■ Sports Stresses (p.142).

Prognosis Depends on the problem. Long-term prevention depends on understanding the causes of the problem and what you can do about them.

Trauma

The neck is vulnerable to a variety of injuries, but the most frequent cause is in car crashes. Cases where there is no fracture, but which are nonetheless severe, are called 'whiplash' injuries.

Symptoms

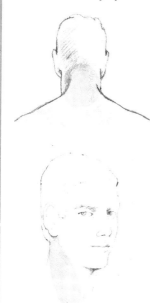

■ If the head is thrown forwards, as in a head-on collision, this will give pain in the back of the neck.

■ If the head is thrown backwards, as in a collision from behind, the muscles and tissues at the front of the neck are overstretched. This is the classic 'whiplash' injury and can cause inability to raise your head off the pillow if you are lying on your back, difficulty in swallowing and jaw tightness.

■ In reality an accident causes the neck to go backwards and forwards. Often all of the neck muscles go into spasm, giving pain all round, which can radiate into the back, arms, head and chest.

■ Shock is one of the main effects. It usually wears off over a few hours or days, but in some cases it can seem to last for months or years. There is also often a degree of concussion, due to the effects on the brain of the rapid acceleration of the head.

■ The effects of such traumas are generally underestimated; the whole body is disrupted. Even in the absence of obvious major injuries, individuals can experience dizziness, low back ache, chest pains, fatigue, poor concentration and lack of confidence.

Treatment

■ Support (p.89).

■ Rest (p.78).

■ Relaxation (p.79).

■ Massage (p.82), once the initial degree of pain diminishes.

■ Sitting Routine (p.112), when your neck feels strong enough.

Prognosis

Most whiplash injuries resolve themselves within a few weeks, but you have to be careful with your neck; the real problem is too much movement, not too little. Occasionally widespread symptoms and delayed shock persist for some time, in which case the help of a qualified therapist is recommended.

Tension Headaches

These arise in the muscles of the neck, scalp and jaw. Muscular tension can also spread to the neck, shoulders and upper back.

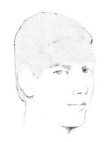

Symptoms

■ Ache usually spreading from the back of the skull, due to tension in the small muscles at the top of the neck. Often gives a tight feeling experienced round the temples and across both sides of the forehead.

■ If the jaw muscles are primarily involved, the ache may be mainly in the face and temples, and can be associated with grinding or clenching of the teeth and clicking in the jaw joints.

■ Your neck may be tense and stiff.

■ It may be associated with symptoms such as giddiness and lack of concentration.

■ The symptoms have a variable pattern and can come and go or remain constant. You may notice when stressful, worrying or overtaxing situations bring the symptoms on.

Causes

Often many factors combine together to cause the tension, particularly stress, muscular tension or joint locking in the neck, trauma, eyestrain and emotional problems. Dental problems may also contribute to tension in your jaw.

Treatment

■ Rest (p.78).

■ Relaxation (p.79). Make a point of letting your jaw relax and do not clench or grind your teeth.

■ Massage (p.82).

■ Painkillers or muscle relaxants (see Medicines p.116).

■ Sitting Routine (p.112).

Prevention

■ Posture (p.121).

■ You should also consider having a dental check-up and an eye test.

Prognosis

Short-term relief can be readily obtained using the above methods. Understanding the causes and trying to resolve them is important in the long-term.

Migraine Headaches

(Vascular headaches.) These result from expansion and contraction of blood vessels in the head.

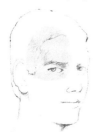

Symptoms

■ Classically the pain is one-sided, principally centred around one temple. However there are other patterns of migraine, where the pain is centred in one eye or is on both sides of the head.

■ The pain is described as bursting or throbbing. It can last from half an hour to several days.

■ It may be associated with giddiness, blurred or distorted vision and be made worse by bright light. Nausea and vomiting may occasionally occur.

■ Neck movements do not affect the pain.

Causes

Susceptible individuals can have migraine triggered by a variety of factors ranging from exertion and relaxation to the contraceptive pill, certain foods, and stress. Tension can be a cause, or result, of migraine; it is important to differentiate between the two. Treatment of the muscular tension may not help to ease the pain.

Treatment

■ Rest (p.78).

■ Relaxation (p.79).

■ If possible lie in a darkened room and sleep it off.

■ Seek the advice of a doctor about the choice and timing of drugs to relieve it; often once a migraine is established it is difficult to relieve.

■ Consider alternative forms of therapy, such as osteopathy, acupuncture or herbal medicines.

Prevention

■ Try to work out the pattern of your migraine and isolate possible triggering factors. If they are caused by relaxing or lying-in at weekends, try to keep up your normal weekday routine.

■ Avoid alcohol and make sure you have a good diet (see Nutrition p.133).

Prognosis

True migraine is difficult to relieve, but if your migraines are severe or frequent, it is worth getting several opinions and trying a variety of alternatives, one of which may work for you.

DIAGNOSIS

Treat Your Problem

This chapter concentrates on the many ways you can treat your back or neck pain. There is also a brief outline of how a qualified therapist will be able to help you. Your problem has probably taken months to develop, so don't expect it to disappear in minutes. If you give your body the right circumstances, however, it can heal even major problems quite quickly.

General Self-Help Treatment

Every individual, and thus every case of back and neck pain, is different, so there is no simple cure that works for every problem. However, as muscular tension is a major cause of back and neck pain, it is important to read this section, no matter what your problem is.

Rest

Rest serves many purposes, the principal ones being:

■ Allowing the body to heal itself. When we rest the nervous and hormonal systems change from being geared towards dynamism and drive to more calm and reparative functions. To recover from any illness you need to rest, and the problems that cause back and neck pain are no exception.

■ Allowing the mind and emotions to wind down. This encourages the healing and relaxation of patterns of body tension and postures. Ideally rest should be combined with Relaxation (p.79).

■ Allowing the muscles to relax to some degree, although this is not the only treatment for muscular problems, as sometimes exercise is more appropriate.

■ Allowing the inflamed tissues to calm down in problems, such as overstretching of the sacro-iliac ligaments or nerve irritation. It is important that a comfortable, well supported position is found, to avoid further strain on the inflamed structures.

Self-Help If your symptoms are not too severe, you can get some rest while carrying on your occupation, by doing things gently, having early nights and resting at the weekends. You don't need to stop everything totally – indeed doing so would make some people more agitated and tense, as they wouldn't know what to do with themselves.

Don't be totally immobile, as movement is a necessary part of your body functions; exercise gently and move about as much as is tolerable, within your own pain limits and without over-exerting yourself. Pain is a way of warning you that you are going too far or doing too much, so take heed of what your body is signalling to you.

Rest is an individual therapy, and what is restful differs between people; holidays are restful for some people and stressful for others. The basic maxim is to do whatever makes you feel good, both mentally and physically. You have to be sensitive to your body's needs. If your problem has been caused by overdoing things, rest might be appropriate; if caused by inactivity, or anxiety, then exercise might be better. Let pain be your guide: if it feels better, carry on; if it makes things worse, don't do it.

Relaxation

The principal aims and effects of relaxation are:

- Releasing the tension in body muscles.

- Quietening the mind.

- Allowing the mind and body to heal, by altering the activity of nerves and hormones.

There are many methods of relaxing, and depths to which one can do it. Most people think of relaxing as just 'switching off', but this is only superficial; effective relaxation is an active process, requiring concentration and effort. Even sleeping is not always relaxing, as can be seen from the number of people who grind their teeth, twist and turn, or wake up tense with aching muscles.

Basic Relaxation Plan　In order to achieve a lasting effect in reducing tension this routine should be practised daily for several weeks, then used when necessary. The secret of relaxation is not to 'try' to relax; it happens as you concentrate on other things.

1　Find a quiet place where you won't be disturbed for about twenty minutes and lie down on a firm, but comfortable, surface. When you get more practised you will be able to do this sitting down, perhaps even in your lunch break at work!

2 Concentrate on breathing slowly and deeply, using your abdominal muscles, and let your mind go still, perhaps visualizing a pleasant image or memory.

3 Concentrate on and contract each of the following muscle groups in turn for five seconds, then relax them for about ten seconds. You should do each side alternately to start with, though eventually you might be able to do both sides together:

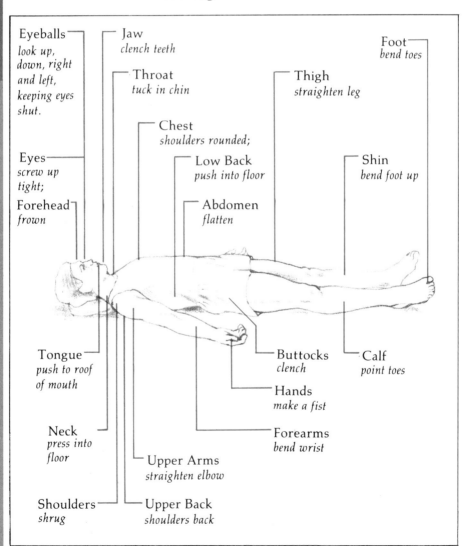

Eyeballs
look up, down, right and left, keeping eyes shut.

Eyes
screw up tight;

Forehead
frown

Jaw
clench teeth

Throat
tuck in chin

Chest
shoulders rounded;

Low Back
push into floor

Abdomen
flatten

Thigh
straighten leg

Foot
bend toes

Shin
bend foot up

Tongue
push to roof of mouth

Neck
press into floor

Shoulders
shrug

Upper Arms
straighten elbow

Upper Back
shoulders back

Buttocks
clench

Hands
make a fist

Forearms
bend wrist

Calf
point toes

4 If you have any pain, outline the area in your mind and identify what shape, size, depth and colour it is; you may find that it changes. Keep trying to pin it down exactly, and when you have it fixed, tense the area for five seconds then let go. Feel it melting away but don't be disappointed if you can't relieve all of it; a slight easing is a good sign and it will all go in time.

5 Become aware of your whole body feeling relaxed. Mentally check over each place in turn; it may feel heavier, bigger, longer, broader or warmer. Enjoy the feeling and visualize peaceful sights, tastes, sounds and sensations. Make a sound if you wish.

As you practice this relaxation and become better at it, you will find that it is difficult to do if you are emotionally upset, angry, or unable to let go of rigid attitudes. Don't be fanatical: stop trying too hard and just let go.

In time you will find that you are able to relax without contracting muscles at all, and more relaxed even when you are not deliberately doing it. Your posture, movements and reactions will become smoother and more comfortable. Your pace of life will become healthier and you will be able to accomplish just as much as when you constantly held yourself tense.

Other Forms of Relaxation

Meditation in its many forms (including many religious processes) is a way of quietening the mind, as are Yoga and Tai Chi. Any physical discipline that involves concentration and effort can, in time, be deeply relaxing; the eastern martial arts aim to achieve this, and it can sometimes be achieved through long-distance running or other individual sports.

You can also try to understand why you are tense and resolve it by changing your attitudes and feelings. This is a difficult process, however, as we rarely see ourselves objectively and are unaware of our subconscious feelings, but you can seek skilled help from a practitioner of one of the many forms of psychotherapy.

Prevention is better than cure, so try to achieve a pace and style of life that doesn't make you increasingly tense. If there is still tension, practice one of the above methods on a regular basis.

Massage

This is one of the most effective methods of relieving pain and sorting out many problems and illnesses throughout the body, not just in the back and neck areas. Massage is rarely harmful and a simple routine is quick to learn; great relief can be given in many cases, even if the person doing it has never done it before.

The Benefits of Massage

Massage has five main effects:

1 Relaxing muscular tension and spasm. As this is the cause of most back and neck problems, relaxing the muscles can relieve most problems and allow the body to resume normal functioning.

2 Breaking down the stringy inelastic muscular fibres, which are caused by chronic contraction. These fibres can be painful, in which case the condition is called fibrositis. This is a bad name as it tends to imply that there is something present other than tight muscle.

3 Stimulating the larger nerve fibres in muscles, which travel to the spinal cord and the skin and inhibit signals from the smaller pain fibres. This is why 'rubbing it better' actually works and reduces the level of pain felt. This effect can be enhanced by the use of irritant rubs, heat creams and embrocations that stimulate the nerves. Irritant poultices, such as a mustard poultice, are still used by some people.

4 Encouraging the circulation, not only in the skin, but also in the deeper structures supplied by related nerves. In this way deeper structures can be affected, as good circulation helps healing, reduces congestion and protects against infection. Massaging the back can help the circulation around the joints and discs; massaging the chest can help the lungs; massaging the stomach can help to relieve colic and wind.

5 Soothing your mind and emotions, just by having somebody else touching you.

Simple Massage Techniques

Self-massage is difficult, as it is hard to relax and do something at the same time. Also the areas that are painful are often hard to reach. It is best to get somebody else to do it for you, but if that is impossible try some of the techniques outlined below as best as you can.

If you are giving a massage, the golden rules are as follows:

■ Do not cause pain. If you find a place that is very tender, back off and work very gently and slowly, and gradually the pain will ease. Trained and experienced therapists sometimes cause pain in order to relieve a problem, but it takes skill to know when to do this. As a general rule, it is better to avoid causing pain.

■ Work slowly and sensitively. Don't just pummel the back, as this will cause the muscles to tense further, as a protective reflex. The purpose of massage is to ease the muscles, not to aggravate them. Listen to what the patient says – if it is too sore he will tell you.

■ Try to relax yourself and your hands while you are doing it, as this will help you to be more sensitive to the places that need working on. The muscles that need attention feel hard and stringy, and you may feel tender iumps. As you work on the muscles, however, they gradually soften, relax and are no longer feel tender; when this happens you should either stop or work on another area.

■ Do not expect to be an expert masseuse at once. It is a skill that takes time, patience and sensitivity to learn. With a little practice, however, you will be able to give relief in a great number of cases of back and neck pain.

■ If there are any nerve symptoms, such as numbness or pins and needles in the arms or legs, ask the patient to keep you informed of how they are; if they worsen, stop and ask the patient to get into a position where they ease again. Always be very gentle where nerves are involved (fortunately this is not very often) and seek expert advice if possible.

Low Back and Thoracic Area Massage

Self-massage is difficult for this area. The masseuse will find the following effective:

1 The patient should be stripped to the waist and lying face down on a firm surface, such as a padded table, a firm bed or the floor. It is important that the patient is comfortable, so place a pillow under the stomach, or anywhere else that he needs. To prevent the neck getting stiff in this position, make sure that he turns his head to face the other way every few minutes.

Simple Massage Position

It is important that the patient is relaxed during massage. A pillow under the stomach can make the low back more comfortable. If you are giving a massage, make sure that you are comfortable and relaxed yourself.

2 Use some oil to ease the movement on the skin, so that it is not irritated; this is particularly important on sensitive skins. Oil can be any sort, even cooking oil. Put a little on the area that you are working and smooth it around.

3 Start at the end of the spine furthest away from the pain and gradually work your way towards it; it will start to relax before you get there.

4 For a general soothing massage use long strokes rubbing over the surface of the oiled skin. To relieve more specific painful nodules or contracted fibres, work with shorter strokes, sometimes just using your thumb and trying to get behind the fibres to stretch them. On the whole the muscles in the back run lengthways, so to stretch them, you should get to the side of them and move across. Just pushing gently into tender muscles can get them to relax.

5 Make sure that you work on the whole of the back and both sides of the spine, even if the symptoms are just on one side.

Thoracic Area In problems associated with the ribs, the muscles in the side and front of the chest may need working on. This should be done with the patient lying on his side or back. In the front of the chest it is usually only the upper ribs and muscles that are tight, so these can be worked on even in women. Massaging the breast tissue should be avoided, as it is sensitive.

Hip, Buttock and Legs In these problems you may need to work on the muscles in the buttock and thigh; this can be done with the patient lying face down, though some are best worked on with the patient on his side or back.

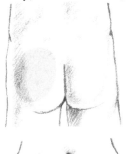

Sacro-iliac ligament problems are often associated with contraction of the muscles that rotate the pelvic bone forward on the painful side. To counteract this, after working on the muscles in the low back, you need to work on the following muscles:

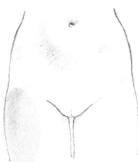

■ Small buttock muscles. A firm thumb pressure to the tight, tender muscle for thirty seconds and repeat if necessary.

■ Muscles at the front of the pelvis. With the patient lying on his back, gently massage with a circular motion for three minutes. The patient can do this themselves if they wish. This should be done each evening or two weeks, combined with the Mild Routine (p.96).

Side Massage Position

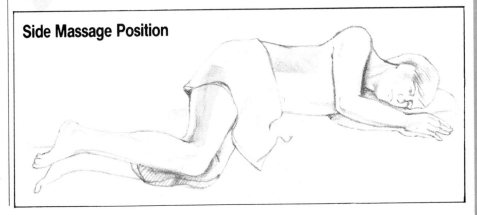

Piriformis syndrome can also be relaxed by firm thumb pressure to the small buttock muscles for two or three minutes until they relax.

Leg pain, if not due to nerve irritation, is likely to be caused by muscular tension down the outside of the thigh. This can be worked on with the patient lying on the non-painful side with a pillow between his knees. Put some oil on the skin and work up the thigh using short strokes of reasonable firmness from both your thumbs. The patient should feel that the muscles relax and become less tender within five minutes.

Neck and Upper Back Massage

The patient can work on this area easily himself, using the fingertips to massage across the muscles from the base of the skull to the top of the back. This can be done in slow, even strokes with one or both hands.

This area is often more difficult to work on for the inexperienced masseuse; in cases of acute spasm in the neck the patient usually cannot turn the neck sufficiently to lie face down, so the masseuse has to work in different positions. The following sequence is usually effective:

1   Get the patient to sit on a stool or sideways on a chair, facing a table on which some firm cushions are placed. The patient should fold his arms and rest them on the cushions, then rest his forehead on his arms. The patient should try to relax in this position, take some deep breaths, and let his head and shoulders 'go heavy' as much as he can.

2   You should work gently into the muscles at the base of the neck and across the shoulders, paying particular attention to trying to soften any stringy, hard or tender muscles. Press gently on any tender places with your thumb for a minute and they will often relax and feel better.

3   Work gently up the neck, but be careful not to put too much force on it, as it is often very sensitive. Increase the relaxation and circulation in the muscles by putting warm towels across the base of the neck; soak a flannel in hot water and wring it out a little, taking care not to burn the skin.

Neck Massage Position

This position is generally safe and comfortable for anyone with tension in the neck and upper back.

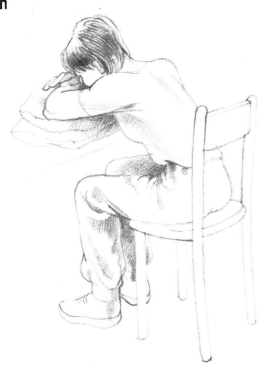

It is important that the height of the table allows the patient to relax and take the full weight of the head on folded arms: use one or two pillows as necessary for comfort. The patient can then concentrate on breathing slowly and deeply using the abdominal muscles.

If you are giving a massage, you should work slowly and gently on the muscles of the upper back and neck.

4   Next get the patient to lie on his back on a firm but comfortable surface and put a couple of pillows or small cushions under the back of his head, so that the back of the neck is slightly stretched. Put your fingers under the back of the neck and gently soothe the tight muscles with slow stroking movements.

5   Finally, gently push your fingertips into the muscles at the very top of the back of the neck, where it joins the skull. If you find any tender lumps, press on them for a few minutes while the patient relaxes. Carry on until the whole of the neck is relaxed and the muscles feel softer. Don't expect all the symptoms to go at once; if you have eased them even a little, you will have broken the pain-spasm-pain reflex, and the problem should get better. You can leave the patient in this position and he can concentrate on Relaxation (p.79) and Breathing (p.135).

Specific Self-Help Treatments

Bedrest

This is particularly recommended for acute low back problems and disc herniation, as it takes the weight off the spine and allows the discs to mend themselves. A true disc problem will only recover, if it is not stressed by the body's weight being transmitted through it.

Self-Help
■ Lie flat on your back or side; sitting propped-up in bed is a bad position as it strains the back. The bed should be firm but not too hard and you may find it more comfortable to use a pillow under your knees when lying on your back, or between your knees when on your side. Do not lie face down (see Sleeping p.131).

■ Get up as infrequently as you can. Eat your meals in bed, if possible, and use a bottle or a bedpan, instead of getting up to go to the toilet. Organize plenty of things to keep your mind occupied, as boredom can lead to low spirits and delay healing.

Treatment for a Typical Disc Problem
■ Total bedrest for three to ten days. When the worst symptoms start to ease do the Mild Routine (p.96), combined with Massage (p.82) and Traction (p.92).

■ If your back is feeling better and the nerve symptoms have eased, get up for a few hours, gradually increasing the time each day. If your back aches, lie on the floor in the Basic Position (see p.97) or with your knees and feet up on a chair.

■ Be careful with sitting, avoid driving if possible, and do not lift anything or bend forwards for at least six weeks.

Undesirable Side-Effects
■ If muscles are not used they will become weaker, especially over a prolonged period of two weeks or more. Bones can also become weak, but take longer, except in elderly people, when they

can be weak already (see Aging p.149). Do the Mild Routine in bed and don't exert yourself after you have been in bed for some time. Get up for only half a day at first, gradually increasing the time as you get stronger.

■ Damaged and healing tissues tend to stiffen up if they are immobilised. In the case of healing tissues, the direction of the fibres of a scar can be haphazard, unless some movement is allowed, to encourage them to align in the right direction. Again, gentle movements while lying down can help this.

Support

There are three main purposes for supporting an area of the low back or neck:

1 To stabilize an area where the muscles or ligaments are weak.

2 To prevent movement, when this might cause damage or pain.

3 To give reassurance to someone who is afraid that the damaged area is too weak to be used without support.

Low Back Area

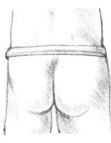
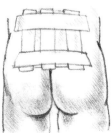

■ Sacro-iliac ligament problems will benefit from stabilizing the pelvis by wearing a sacro-iliac belt, available from drugstores or specialist shops. This should be tight fitting and worn below the bony prominences at the front and back of the pelvis. It can be used until the pain eases and as a preventative measure during strenuous activity. It should not be worn during pregnancy.

■ Disc herniation may be helped by strapping the back with wide strips of adhesive plaster. The sensation of this stretching as you bend forward is a warning against unguarded movements. It may irritate the skin and can be difficult to get off – try soaking in a hot bath first.

■ In acute cases general support for the low back is usually given by means of a corset. In the long-term these can be unnecessary and potentially harmful, as dependence on them causes the normally active supporting muscles to weaken.

They can only be justified if the trunk or low back muscles have been weakened by a disease, such as polio, or an operation. Otherwise the muscles should be strengthened by exercise and any excess weight should be lost.

■ Heavy lifting can be made safer and easier by wearing a strong belt around the waist, which helps the stomach muscles to support the back. It is an aid rather than a substitute for strong muscles, but if your work involves a great deal of heavy lifting, you should consider using one of these.

Neck Area In an emergency, if your neck is locked in an awkward position, you may get some relief from a temporary collar. This be made by folding several sheets of newspaper to the same width as the length of your neck and tying them round your neck with a light woollen scarf. A towel wrapped round the neck will also provide short-term relief.

Severe problems can be helped by the use of a manufactured light collar, made from polystyrene, sponge or plastic. The drawback is that this can become a substitute for really sorting out your neck problem with proper treatment. Trauma, however, may require the neck to be supported for a week or more, especially if the ligaments are injured.

Heat

Heat causes the small blood vessels and capillaries to dilate, increasing the flow of blood into an area and improving the circulation and drainage. This can also have an effect on deeper structures via the nerves; lung, intestinal and pelvic problems can often be eased by warming the area over them. Muscles respond best of all to this treatment, as the application of heat improves the flow of blood, relieves the pain and relaxes the muscle.

Self-Help In an emergency or if you cannot move, heat can be effectively applied to the lower back using hot towels or a hot water bottle. Hot towels can also be easily wrapped round the neck. Otherwise heat can be applied according to your personal preference or the limitations of your situation.

■ A soak in a hot bath, a sauna or a shower can relax the muscles generally. This is particularly useful if you are aching in many areas and it also combines the benefits of rest and relaxation.

■ You can apply heat to a more specific area using a hot water bottle or an electric heat pad, available from your drugstore. Infra-red lamps can also be used, although they can be more awkward to position.

■ You need to apply heat for at least fifteen minutes for it to achieve the full effect. This will be increased by rest and relaxation and, once the muscles have begun to relax, gentle exercise. Take care not to burn yourself from excessive heat.

■ You can also use your own body heat to help yourself, by wrapping up warmly. A scarf around the neck can ease neck pains, while a thermal vest or towel wrapped round the waist can ease low back aches. If you keep moving and keep warm when in a cold environment, you should have good circulation in your muscles and little chance of aches.

Ice

Cold makes the capillaries constrict and reduces the flow of blood, which can be useful immediately after an injury, such as a bruise or an overstretched ligament following a blow or a fall, to prevent too much inflammation and swelling. It should not be used once the injury has calmed down and is beginning to heal. Compression, or applying pressure to the area, helps the ice to prevent swelling.

In more chronic inflammations, such as those associated with some forms of arthritis, ice can ease the inflammation. It should not be used for long periods, however, otherwise ill-effects from the decreased circulation may appear; two minutes is usually sufficient.

Alternately bathing in hot and cold water has been advocated as a stimulant to the circulation for many centuries. It is probably effective, as the body needs stimulation to function at its best. On a cold day it is better to wrap up warm and go outside for a brisk walk, rather than stay inside in a stuffy atmosphere, encouraging congestion.

Cold can make the muscles tense so don't use it in cases of muscular tension.

Traction

Traction stretches the spine lengthways to separate the vertebrae and take pressure off the discs, thus reducing any bulging and helping them to heal.

Disc herniation, in particular, responds well to this treatment. This problem takes a long time to heal fully, but temporary relief can be obtained using the first three methods below.

Bedrest Traction Lie on your back with your legs out straight and with your arms resting beside you on the bed. Ask a friend to grip hold of your ankles and pull lengthways and slightly upwards. The force required is not great, but it should be sufficient to stretch your back, without pulling you down the bed. Too much force does not do more good, and in some cases excessive force can be counter-productive. To protect your friend's back, get him to apply the traction by leaning backwards with straight arms. The traction should be applied for about thirty seconds, then relaxed for thirty seconds, and repeated ten times. This can be done several times a day.

Bedrest Traction

Traction while the patient is confined to bed can provide additional relief in cases of disc herniation. The force applied should only be moderate and the person applying the traction should take care not to injure their own back.

Hanging Traction This can be done from anything that is strong enough to take your weight, and convenient for you to get a good grip on such as the top of a door (near the hinges) or a secure metal bar. Stretch up, grip the bar, keeping your arms straight, and bend your knees to let yourself hang. Let your back relax while you are doing this, and if you feel confident, take your feet off the ground completely. Do this for thirty seconds and repeat as above.

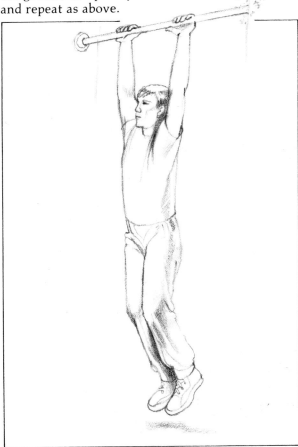

Neck Traction Some cases of nerve irritation in the neck area can be treated with traction.

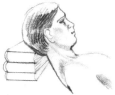

Lie on a firm surface and rest your head on about 12 cm (5 in) of books, with the edge of the books just under the base of your skull, where it joins your neck. Tuck in your chin and relax your shoulders. This will provide a stretching and traction force. It is also a good position to relax in.

Leg Swinging In some cases of piriformis syndrome and hip joint problems, this exercise can exert a traction effect.

Stand on a low stool or the bottom step of a flight of stairs with your good leg and hold on to a firm support with the hand of your good side. Let the painful leg swing freely. Concentrate on relaxing the whole leg and let it become heavy, so that its weight exerts a mild traction effect.

Start with small arcs of swing and build up gradually, without forcing it further than is comfortable; keep your back still. If you find that you can do this comfortably, swing the leg like a pendulum across your body for as long as you feel comfortable; five to ten minutes is generally enough. If both hips are stiff, repeat the exercise with the other leg. Do at least once a day.

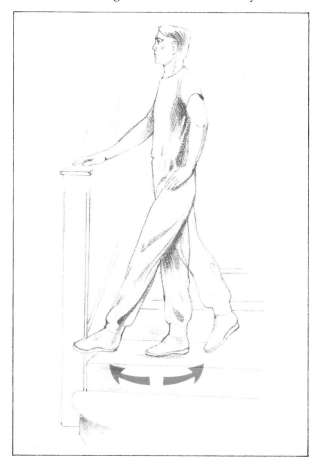

Therapeutic Exercises

This section is concerned with specific therapeutic exercises for your back and neck, with three principal aims:

1 To improve the strength and tone of muscles.

2 To stretch tight or shortened tissues.

3 To improve the circulation in and relax muscles.

Using the Routines

The exercise routines can be used as a measure of your fitness. If you have difficulty with a particular exercise, this tells you that those muscles need attention, so persevere with the exercise until you can do it easily. You will then be able to progress to the next routine. For convenience and safety the exercises have been grouped into four routines. The first three routines are designed to be added on to each other, so for each routine you should run through the preceding ones first.

Mild Routine This is the only routine to be used if you are suffering from:

■ any condition requiring bedrest;

■ an illness;

■ a major trauma;

■ disc herniation;

■ nerve irritation;

■ acute sacro-iliac ligament problems;

■ excess weight and have not exercised regularly for over three months.

In this routine all the exercises are done lying down, so it is safe for almost any problem at any age, even if you are resting in bed. Do not attempt either of the other routines until you have recovered and become fitter, and have done this routine every day for two weeks.

Intermediate Routine This routine can be done only if:

- you have done the Mild Routine for at least two weeks;
- you do not have any of the problems listed above;
- the Mild Routine does not aggravate your symptoms.

Vigorous Routine This is an optional routine, as basic back and neck fitness can be maintained on the Mild and Intermediate Routines. You should do this routine only if:

- you have done the Intermediate Routine daily for three weeks;
- the Intermediate Routine does not aggravate your symptoms;
- you do not have any of the problems listed above.

If you are elderly, or in doubt, ask the opinion of a qualified therapist before doing this routine.

Sitting Routine This is primarily for neck and thoracic area problems, as sitting can aggravate low back area problems. It is ideal for people who have sedentary occupations and it can be done at any time during the day. It should be combined with one of the other routines when you have the time.

Frequency of Routines As a therapeutic measure these routines should be done once a day, preferably not first thing in the morning, as your muscles tend to be stiffer and your discs more vulnerable at this time. If you are basically fit, do the routines twice a day if you have time, but be careful not to overdo it.

Mild Routine

Do not rush any of the exercises, even if they seem easy; it takes time for your body to change. For some exercises there is a description of how to make the exercise stronger. This should only be done if you are basically fit or have been doing the routine for at least a week.

Basic Position Lie down and flatten your low back against the floor, by bending your knees up to forty-five degrees, with your feet flat on the floor. Flattening your spine in this way is called the Pelvic Tilt (p.123). Check to see if your low back is flat against the floor by trying to slide your hand under it. This is the Basic Position and is the starting point for many of the exercises. This position is safe to lie in and is usually comfortable whatever your back problem.

The Pelvic Tilt must be maintained throughout all the exercise routines, in order to protect your back, strengthen your abdominal muscles and improve your posture. Keep your chin tucked in and your neck lengthened.

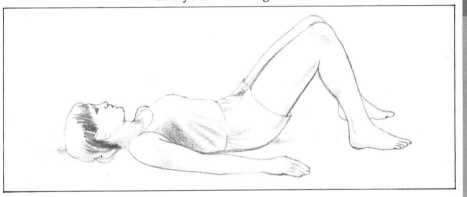

Relaxation This must be done before and after each sequence of exercises, and during them if you are doing one routine after another:

1 Let your mind relax and breathe slowly and deeply, using your abdominal muscles.

2 Clench your arms and fists tight, then let them relax.

3 Shrug your shoulders up, hold for five seconds, then relax.

4 Clench your toes and calves tight, then let them relax.

5 Clench your buttocks tight, then let them relax.

Breathing and Concentration Concentrate on breathing deeply and slowly into your abdomen (see Breathing p.135). Breathe out fully with the upper chest, then let it rest and just use your diaphragm and abdominal muscles. Time the exercises so that the exertion occurs as you breathe out; rest as you breathe in. Focusing your attention on your whole body during the exercises will help to unwind the subconscious patterns of tension in both your mind and body.

Low Back Stretch This stretches and relaxes the low back and buttock muscles. Start in the Basic Position and bend both knees up together so that you can clasp your hands round them. Do not pull hard, just let them rest naturally for a moment. Keep your head down and pull gently with your arms until your low back begins to stretch or lift slightly off the floor. Hold it there and take a deep breath. As you breathe out let your back relax and stretch further. Hold this stretched position for five seconds then relax. Repeat five times.

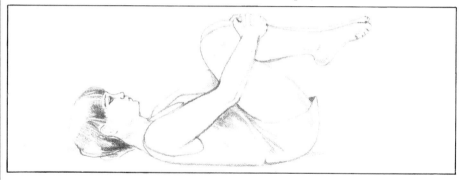

Hip Flexor Stretch Start in the Basic Position and lift one leg up, with the knee bent, so that you can clasp it with both hands. Pull it up to your chest and hold it there; slide the other leg out straight and stretch it, without letting your back arch. Hold for five seconds. Do this with the opposite leg and repeat five times.

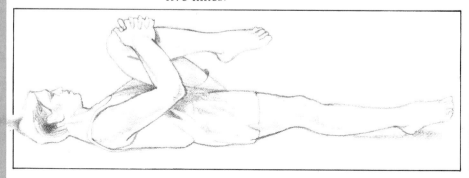

Cross Arm-Leg Push This strengthens the stomach muscles. Start in the Basic Position and bend one leg up slightly. Put the opposite hand on it near the knee with your arm out straight. As you breathe out, push your leg and arm together quite firmly and hold for five seconds. Relax and take a deep breath. Repeat the exercise five times, then do it with the other leg and arm.

Stronger exercise: Do the above with your head held off the ground and chin tucked in.

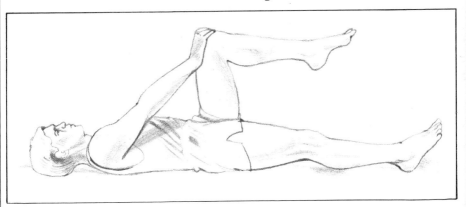

Lateral Leg Lift This strengthens the muscles at the sides of your body. Lie on your side with your body and upper leg in a straight line and your lower leg bent up to ninety degrees. Put your lower arm under your head and the upper arm palm down on the floor balancing your body. Keep your pelvis in the Pelvic Tilt position. Breathe in deeply then slowly lift the upper leg up to thirty degrees and let it down again as you breathe out. Repeat ten times for each side.

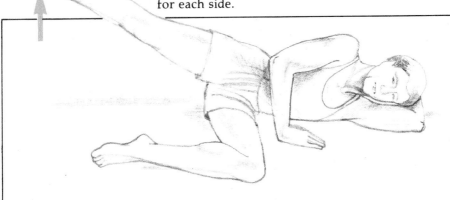

Curl-Up   This strengthens your stomach muscles. Start in the Basic Position and stretch out your arms in front of you. Breathe in and slowly curl your neck and upper back up, as you breathe out, until your fingers can touch the top of your knees. Hold this position for five seconds then lower yourself slowly. Keep your feet and low back flat against the floor. Repeat five times.

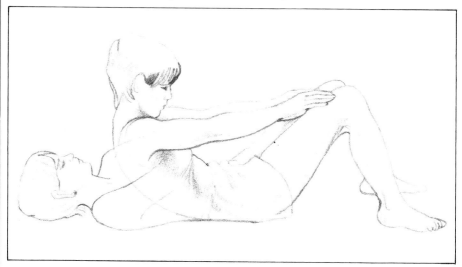

Arm-Leg Stretch   This exercise stretches the muscles down the sides of your body. Lie on your back with your legs straight and your arms outstretched above your head. Breathe in and stretch the arm and leg of one side in opposite directions, as you breathe out, so that your whole side is stretched. Relax and do the same for the other side. Repeat five times. Finally stretch both arms and legs at the same time, keeping your low back flat. Hold for five seconds, then relax.

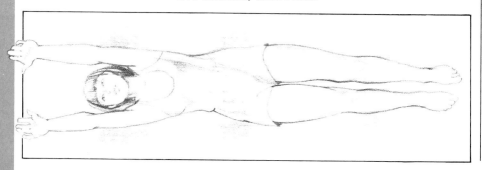

Head Roll This stretches the neck muscles. Lie on your back in any comfortable position, with your arms by your side. Tuck your chin in and lengthen your neck. Breathe in deeply and let your head turn to one side as you breathe out. Do not force it – just let the weight of your head take it there. Hold for five seconds, let your head turn a little further, then return to your starting position. Repeat for each side five times.

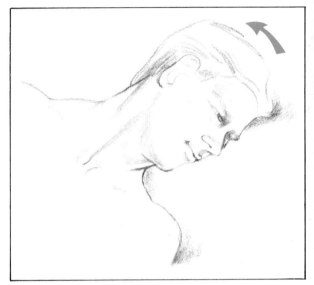

Relaxation As described above. Lie on your back in any position that is comfortable, not forgetting the Pelvic Tilt. In the Basic Position you may be able to relax more easily if you put pillows under your knees or rest your lower legs on a low chair or bed. Stay relaxed for as long as you wish.

Let your body unwind and your mind quieten. Breathe deeply and enjoy the good feeling. Do not underestimate the importance of relaxation both before and after exercise; you need to be able to relax to stay healthy. Exercise on its own is not enough; even determined exercise fanatics can collapse because they overstress themselves. Exercise done without relaxation can be counter-productive.

If you are moving on to the Intermediate Routine, relax for two to five minutes, do the Intermediate Routine and then relax for longer at the end.

Intermediate Routine

Don't forget to breathe out as you carry out a movement or contraction and maintain the Pelvic Tilt Position at all times. Do the Mild Routine first.

Double Lateral Leg Lift This strengthens the muscles of your side. Lie on your side as for the Single Lateral Leg Lift but with both legs straight. Raise both legs off the floor slightly; hold the lower one and raise the upper leg and let it down again slowly. Let both legs down. Repeat five times for both sides.

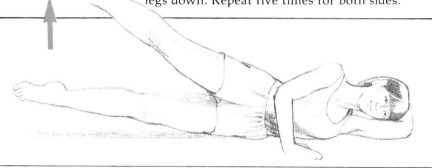

Bicycling This strengthens your stomach muscles. Lie on your back in the Basic Position, keeping your back flat and knees bent. Raise your feet off the floor and move your legs as if you were riding a bicycle. Keep this up for about fifteen seconds. Rest and repeat three times. Don't forget to breathe in and out while you are doing it.

Stronger exercise: Stretch your legs out horizontally as you bicycle, which uses the abdominal muscles even more.

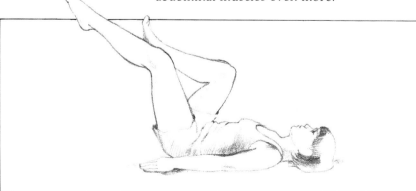

Hamstring Stretch   This exercise should not be done if you have any nerve symptoms, such as pins and needles or numbness, in your legs. Start in the Basic Position and straighten one leg fully, keeping the knee locked; bend your toes towards your head to stretch your calf. Lift the leg up as far as you can, until you feel the muscles at the back of your thigh stretching. Return to the starting position and do the same with the other leg. Repeat five times for each leg.

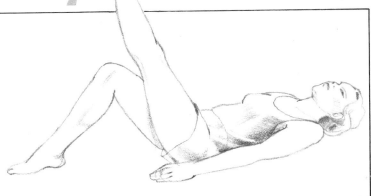

Stronger Hip Flexor Stretch   Miss out this exercise if you do not have a bed available. Lie in the Basic Position on the edge of a bed. Clasp the inner leg to your chest and let the outer leg drop over the edge of the bed as you breathe out. Hold for five seconds. Repeat five times then do the same with the other leg on the other side of the bed.

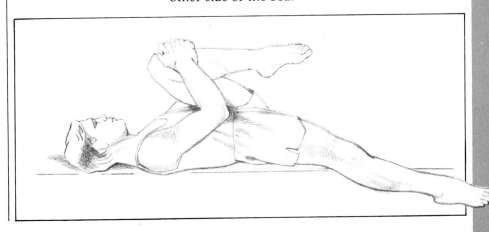

Sit-Down This strengthens the stomach muscles and improves your ability to maintain the Pelvic Tilt Position in a variety of positions. Start in the Basic Position and use your arms to push yourself up to a sitting position. Take a deep breath in and let your spine curl down towards the floor as you exhale, until you are lying flat. Keep your feet on the floor and your arms outstretched throughout the movement. Let your spine down slowly, so that each vertebra meets the floor in turn. Repeat five times, but stop if your back hurts.

Stronger exercise: Do this exercise with your arms folded.

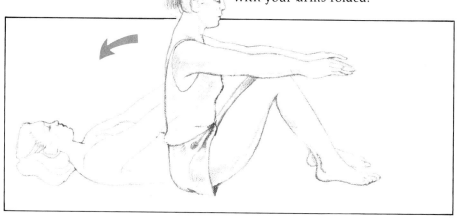

Cat Back This improves general mobility and coordination. Turn over so that you are on all fours, with your hands and knees slightly apart. Breathe in and arch your back upwards as you breathe out, letting your head drop towards the floor. Stretch, relax and breathe in again. As you breathe out, arch your back down towards the floor and pull your head back. Stretch for a few seconds then relax. Repeat five times.

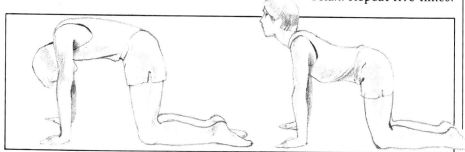

Cat Stretch   This stretches the front of your chest. Starting on all fours, slide your hands forward until you feel the front of your chest stretching, your forehead will be nearly touching the floor. Stretch then return to the starting position. Repeat five times.

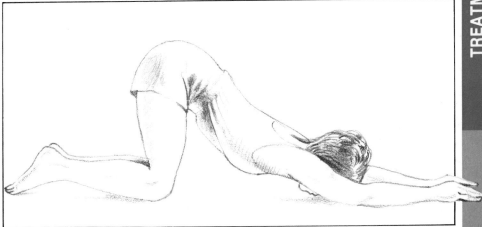

Relaxation   As for the Mild Routine. If you are moving on to the Vigorous Routine, relax for two to five minutes, do the Vigorous Routine and then relax for longer at the end.

Vigorous Routine

This should only be done if your spine is relatively healthy, and you have done the Mild Routine for two weeks, followed by the Intermediate Routine for three weeks. If any exercise causes sharp back pains, stop and return to the other routines until your back is stronger.

As the exercises are now getting more time consuming, you do not need to do this routine every day, but should do it at least twice a week to keep your back healthy.

Do the Mild Routine and the Intermediate Routine first, to make sure that you are fully warmed up and relaxed. You must maintain the Pelvic Tilt position throughout these exercises to protect your back.

Arm Circles This exercise stretches your shoulder muscles. Stand with your feet comfortably apart and your arms by your sides. Cross your arms in front of you slowly as you breathe in deeply. Carry on with your arms until they are above your head, at which point you can start to breathe out. Bring your arms downwards and backwards to your sides, stretching the front of your chest. Try to do this in one smooth movement. Repeat five times.

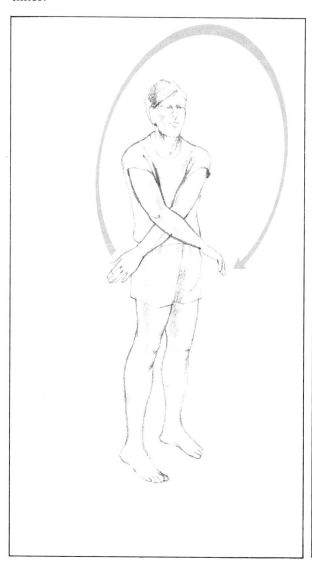

Chest Stretch Stand comfortably, clasping your hands together behind your back. Keeping your arms straight, breathe in and lift them up until they are as high as they can go – usually mid-back height. Hold for a few seconds then relax. Repeat five times.

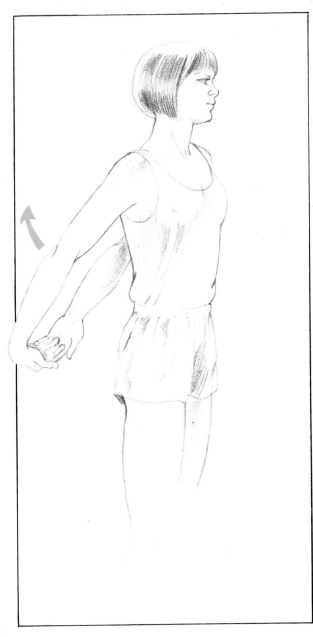

Side Bend This stretches the sides of your body. Stand, with your feet apart, in the Pelvic Tilt position. Stretch one arm up and slowly bend towards the other side, while exhaling, by sliding your hand down your leg. Don't twist or bend forwards as you do this. Return to the starting position and do the same to the other side. Repeat five times for each side.

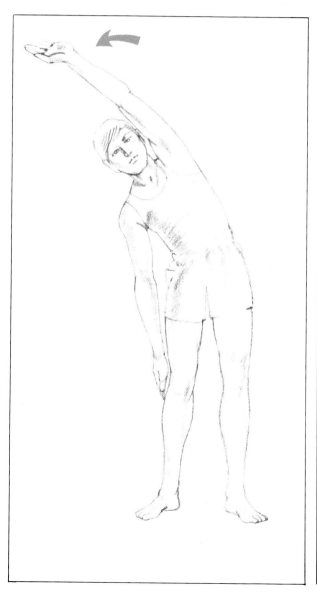

Toe Touch This is a good test of basic back health and flexibility: if you can do it without discomfort, your back is fairly strong; if it causes pain, you should return to the Intermediate Routine.

Stand with your feet comfortably apart keeping your legs straight. Curl slowly forwards until your torso is hanging down, with your arms stretched towards the floor. Take a deep breath, breathe out, relax and stretch a bit further. Hang for a few seconds then slowly straighten up. Repeat three times. Do not worry if you cannot touch the floor yet; you will be able to if you practice this frequently.

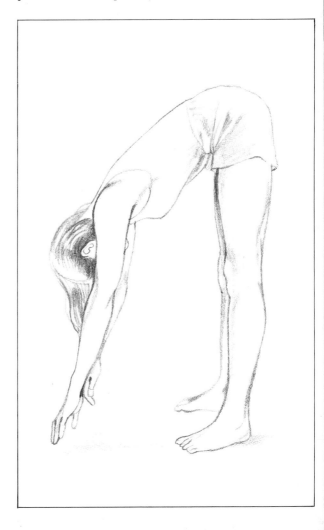

Sit-Up This strengthens the stomach muscles and improves the muscular control of your low back. Start in the Basic Position with your arms outstretched in front of you; breathe in and curl slowly upwards as you breathe out, until you are sitting. Breathe in again and lower yourself while breathing out. Repeat five times.

It is important to keep your knees bent and your feet flat on the floor during this exercise, and to do it smoothly, without jerking your body up or letting it crash down.

Stronger exercise: Do it with your arms folded across your chest or, more difficult still, clasped behind your head.

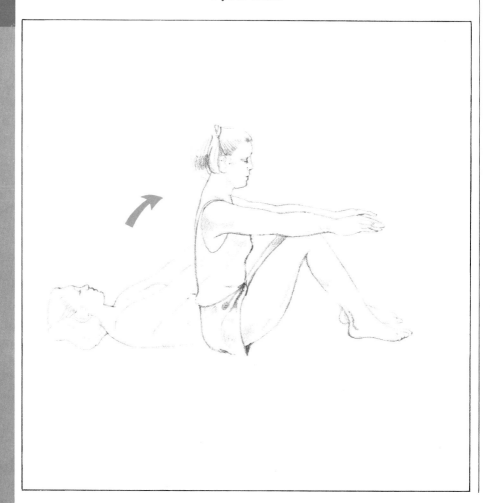

Sitting Hamstring Stretch Sit upright on the floor with your legs out in front of you. Pull one foot towards you and place the sole of it against the opposite knee. Curl your body forwards slowly, and stretch your arms towards the ankle of the straight leg. When you feel your thigh muscles stretch, take a deep breath; breathe out and stretch a little further. Hold for a few seconds then relax. Repeat five times for each leg.

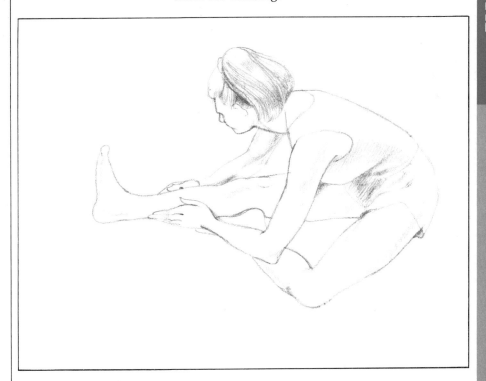

Relaxation As for the Mild Routine. Relax as long as you like.

Sitting Routine

This routine aims to improve the function of the neck and upper back. It can be done anywhere while sitting down (especially at a desk), but you must have an upright chair with a firm seat, not a soft armchair. It should be done at least once every working day; if you are sitting all day, do it at least twice (mid-morning and mid-afternoon).

Once you have learnt to use this exercise routine and to relax quickly, you will find that you feel refreshed after it; rather than losing work time, you will be able to work more effectively because you feel better in yourself.

Prolonged sitting may aggravate low back problems. The Mild Routine is more suitable for these cases.

Sitting Position Sit upright with your feet on the floor and hands resting on your lap. Improve your posture with the Pelvic Tilt position (p.123): flatten your low back by using your abdominal muscles and let your pelvic bones sink into the chair (even if it is hard). Lengthen your spine further with the Neck Lengthening position (p.123). Let your shoulders drop down and broaden out.

Relaxation This can be done as for the Mild Routine (see p.96), but in the Sitting Position.

Breathing and Concentration Concentrate on breathing slowly and deeply into your abdomen (see Breathing p.135). Breathe out fully with the upper chest, then let it rest and just use your diaphragm and abdominal muscles. Time the exercises so that the exertion occurs as you breathe out; rest as you breathe in.

Abdominal Strengthening This exercise strengthens your abdominal muscles and helps your breathing. Start in the Sitting Position and give your muscles an extra hard contraction when you breathe out; hold this for two seconds then relax and breathe in. Repeat three times.

Put the palms of your hands onto your knees; as you breathe out, push your hands and knees together as hard as you can. Hold this for three seconds and repeat three times.

Head Roll This stretches the neck muscles. Turn your head slowly in one direction as if you were looking over your shoulder. Keep your upper back and shoulders facing forwards. When you get to the limit of the movement (don't force it), take a deep breath in; as you breathe out let your head turn a bit further. Hold for a second then return to the starting position. Repeat three times in each direction.

Shoulder Circles This loosens the shoulder muscles. Shrug both your shoulders right up towards your ears; hold for a second, then drop them down. Pull your shoulders backwards as far as they will go; hold for a second, then relax. Push your shoulders forwards as far as you can; hold for a second, then relax.

Repeat these three steps three times then finish off by doing three smooth circles, following the steps above. If you feel adventurous, do three circles in the opposite direction.

Chest Stretch This opens out your chest. Clasp your hands together behind your back, and behind your chair if it has a low back; raise them up as high as you can, keeping them clasped. When you get to the limit of your movement (without forcing it), take a deep breath in; as you breathe out, lift your arms a little higher then relax. Repeat twice.

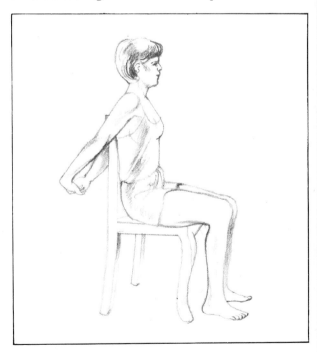

Upper Back Stretch This improves the mobility of the upper thoracic area. Clasp your hands behind your neck, fingers interlaced. Position them so that they are holding the base rather than the top of your neck. Pull your elbows as near together as you can. Twist round to one side as you breathe out and hold for a second; breathe in and then twist to the other side as you breathe out. Repeat five times each way.

Each time you do this you can alter the focus of the stretch by bending your head and neck forwards a bit more. Do not bend so far that you start to twist your low back. Once you have mastered this, you will be able to concentrate on stretching any tight muscles by the right combination of forward bending and twisting.

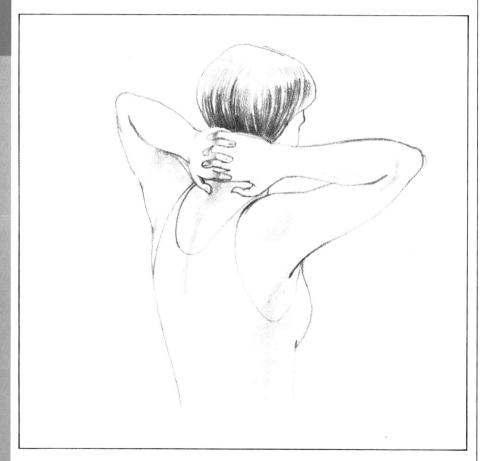

Arm Reaches These loosen the shoulder muscles. Start with your hands resting in your lap. Lift up one arm and point it out straight in front of you. Breathe in and push it further forwards as you breathe out. Don't twist your spine – keep facing forwards. Do this twice more, then let the arm drop and repeat for the other arm.

Lift the first arm up so that it is pointing vertically. Hold it there, breathe in and push it further upwards as you breathe out. Repeat three times with each arm. Finally lift both arms into the air; push upwards and hold for three seconds, then relax.

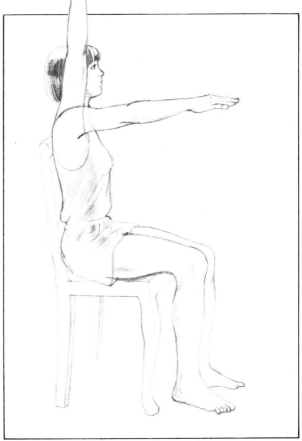

Self-Massage Lift one hand up onto the opposite shoulder and use your fingers to work into the tight muscles of your neck and upper back. If you feel a tender spot, push onto it gently for a few seconds. Don't forget to keep breathing, even if it is painful. Do this for a minute or so each side.

Relaxation As for the Mild Routine (p.96).

Medicines and Professional Treatment

Medicines

There are many types of medicines that can be used in the treatment of back and neck problems. The majority of these are aimed at symptomatic relief, which is treating the effects rather than the causes, and thus have limited value in getting you better.

It is unwise to rely on medicines for the treatment of back and neck problems, especially in the long-term; mechanical or functional problems need mechanical or functional, not chemical, treatment, except when general illness and fatigue are contributing to your problems.

Painkillers Asprin and non-aspirin drugs, available from drugstores or on prescription, can dull mild pain, but are rarely totally effective against severe pain. Stronger narcotic painkillers are available, but carry a risk of addiction.

Anti-Inflammatory Drugs Aspirin and non-aspirin drugs, available from drugstores, and other specific anti-inflammatory drugs are available on prescription from your doctor. They can provide some relief but have several drawbacks, mainly side-effects of nausea and indigestion. Furthermore, they are often ineffective and taken inappropriately. You could consider them in cases of arthritis, sacro-iliac ligament problems and disc herniation.

Muscle Relaxants These are available on prescription from your doctor. In theory they should be effective, as muscles cause most symptoms; in practice, however, they are not very effective; except in an extreme case of muscular spasm when they can break the pain-spasm-pain reflex. As these drugs are usually tranquillizers also, they tend to make you lethargic and can create a drug dependence.

They are useful in a crisis, but you should be wary of taking them in the long-term, as prolonged use carries the danger of withdrawal symptoms.

Herbal Medicines and Homeopathic Remedies These are controversial and as yet their efficacy remains unproven, although the benefits found by many people suggest that they can be beneficial. If you know of a remedy that helps you, by all means take it; it may help you and is unlikely to do any harm, as there are few side-effects from these medicines, if taken as recommended.

Note You should never take more than the dose recommended on the packet or prescribed by your doctor; this applies to all medicines.

Professional Treatment

This section briefly describes some of the approaches to treatment that may be carried out if you consult a qualified therapist. The skill of a good therapist lies not just in what he does, but in his ability to diagnose, understand, reassure and give good advice.

Unfortunately there are many bad therapists in practice, and too few good ones, so it is best to select a therapist either by personal recommendation from a friend or by enquiring from professional organizations. Be sure to see the practitioner for at least fifteen minutes. In some cases it takes up to an hour to get to grips with a problem properly.

Manipulation This is a bad name as manipulation really means using the hands to treat, thus it includes massaging and gentle releasing manoevres. It has, however, come to be accepted to mean the high velocity 'clicking' of joints, mainly in the spine. The purpose of a high velocity click is to break the reflex of muscular spasm that can hold a joint locked. In trained hands it can be a very effective form of treatment, especially for acute joint locking.

In some quarters it has come to be regarded as a panacea for all back and neck problems, which is unfortunate; indeed manipulation can make many problems, such as disc herniation, nerve irritation and sacro-iliac ligament problems, worse, and is dangerous in cases where the bone is weak or damaged. Correct diagnosis is essential before manipulation is attempted, and a long and specialized training is necessary, before a practitioner can apply it with minimal strain and trauma to the surrounding tissues.

Stories of the doubled-up patient being cured by one click are true, but this is possible only in a minority of cases. Many osteopaths and chiropractors, who are renowned for being good at manipulating, actually click joints very rarely, as other more gentle skills are often more effective and less traumatic. If you consult a 'manipulative therapist', let him decide what is appropriate in your case, and ask him to explain why.

You should beware of the therapist who repeatedly clicks the same joints without working on your muscles, as this means that he is not sorting out the real problem. Frequently repeated manipulation can lead to joint hypermobility, which is why self-manipulation is inadvisable and should not be attempted.

Some orthopaedic specialists may suggest putting you under a general anaesthetic before manipulating your spine. This is usually unnecessary, though rarely permanently harmful. You might consider getting a second opinion from a skilled manipulator before agreeing to this.

Surgery This is necessary only in a very small percentage of back and neck problems, such as:

- major damage, perhaps from a fracture;

- a massive disc herniation pressing on several nerves;

- when the disc has healed badly leaving a sequestrum;

- in severe spondylolisthesis;

- in the rare occurances of a spinal tumour.

Sometimes surgery is also carried out when a disc does not heal fully and continues to press on a nerve. In an operation called a laminectomy, a piece of the vertebra is cut away and the herniated disc material is removed. This is often successful at relieving the nerve symptoms, but leaves scar tissue, so that the back is sometimes painful afterwards. Vertebrae can also be fused together with a bone graft. The problem with this is that more pressure is put on the vertebrae above.

Surgery is not without its problems, and should be avoided whenever possible, by trying alternative treatments first. It is however necessary in some cases and your back can become healthy again with good post-operative care, massage and regular exercise when it has healed.

Injections These are used by many doctors, who claim to achieve a variety of effects, such as freeing nerve roots, strengthening ligaments and dissolving discs. The results, however, seem unpredictable and unconvincing. Such benefit as can seem to be derived can actually be achieved by just sticking a needle in (like acupuncture), which may help to break a pain-spasm-pain reflex.

There is an argument that supports the use of ligament strengthening injections in chronic sacro-iliac ligament problems, but apart from that, the use of injections should be treated with scepticism and alternative methods should be considered. The self-help methods already described in this chapter are likely to give better results in the majority of cases. Remember that most cases of acute back pain get better within two weeks anyway.

Other Treatments There are many other methods that are used to try to treat back and neck pain, such as Transcutaneous Nerve Stimulation, and various other electrical therapies. The results of these seem discouraging. Anything that helps to relax the muscles is obviously useful, but you are more likely to get relief from heat, rest, relaxation and massage.

Acupuncture does seem to have some benefit in some cases of back and neck pain, especially when used to relieve muscle spasm; if you believe in it, you could consider consulting a trained acupuncturist.

Prevent Your Problem Recurring

*T*he measures outlined in this chapter will not only help previous back and neck pain sufferers, but will also prevent problems developing in healthy spines. The early treatment of minor aches and pains in your back or neck is invaluable in preventing the development of more serious problems: don't ignore these symptoms, especially if they are recurrent.

Posture

Correct posture is vital for the prevention of back and neck pain as postural stresses play a large part in the development of most problems. You should appreciate, however, that it is not always what the posture looks like that is important, it is how well your body is coping with that posture. Few people have ideal curves in their spines; most spines are asymmetrical or unusually curved in some way. That causes no problems unless one of the structures in the spine is under more strain than it can cope with.

Front to Back Posture

Ideal posture depends on the balanced tone of all the supporting muscles, together with the integrity of the bones, discs, joints and ligaments. The most frequently seen pattern of poor or imbalanced posture, involves tight muscles in the low back and neck and slack abdominal muscles. This causes the pelvis to tip forwards, the stomach to stick out, the shoulders to appear rounded, the thoracic area to look stooped and the chin to project forwards. Any excess weight will make this worse. Poor posture places strain on many of the spinal structures and may eventually lead to back problems developing.

Self-Assessment   Look at yourself from the side in a full-length mirror and compare your line of weight-bearing with the ideal plumb-line in the diagram on the next page. Does your posture look bad?

■ Feel the tension in your low back muscles, if they are tight and tender they are overworking.

■ Stand with your heels, buttocks, shoulders and head flat against a wall. If the space between your low back and the wall is more than the flat of your hand, you need to practise the Pelvic Tilt (p.123).

■ Feel the back of your neck with your hand; is it very curved inwards, with tight and compressed muscles? You need to practise Neck Lengthening (p.123).

Test and Improve Your Front to Back Posture

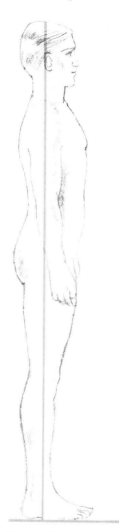

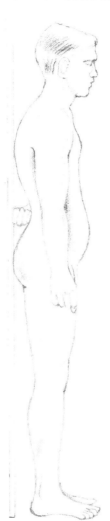

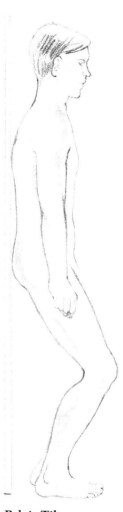

Correct Posture
The ideal plumb-line (above) should align the ear, shoulder, hip and knee. Compare the flat stomach and gentle curves of the back with poor posture (centre).

Poor Posture
Test your posture by standing against a wall: if you can get as much as a fist between your low back and the wall, you need to practise the Pelvic Tilt (right).

Pelvic Tilt
Tighten your stomach muscles and flatten your low back against the wall. This will be easier if you bend your knees, hold your back flat, then straighten them again.

■ To assess the tone and strength of your abdominal muscles, lie on your back, with your knees bent and your feet flat on the ground. With your arms outstretched, lift your body up to a sitting position. Can you do it? If not you need to do the Mild Routine (p.96). The importance of good strength and tone in the abdominal muscles cannot be overemphasized.

■ In acute low back problems you may find that you are bent over or to one side. If this is the case, do not worry or try to force it straight, as it will right itself when the problem has healed.

Pelvic Tilt   This means rotating your pelvis backwards. You can do this by tightening your abdominal muscles, while relaxing your buttock muscles. Try this when standing against a wall and see if you can flatten the space behind your low back. Feel what it should be like by bending your knees slightly, which will flatten your spine. With practice you will also be able to tilt your pelvis backwards and flatten your lumbar spine when you are sitting or lying down. You should consult Sitting Posture (p.125) and practise the Basic Position (p.97).

Neck Lengthening   Tuck in your chin and lengthen your neck, as if it were being pulled upwards by a string. You should feel as if you become slightly taller, especially if you let your whole back lengthen with the Pelvic Tilt. Having started to correctly balance the two ends of your spine, the rest will take care of itself. Let your shoulders drop and open the front of your chest. Balance your weight evenly on your heels and toes. Relax and take some deep breaths in and out, using your abdomen rather than your chest (see Breathing p.135). It will take some time before this posture becomes natural, as changing habits is not easy. Perseverence, however, will help to relieve and prevent most back problems.

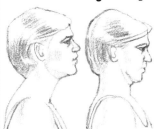

Side to Side Posture

Ideally your body should be symmetrical and your spine straight when viewed from behind. Many people have small degrees of asymmetry, which cause no problems. Don't get carried away or worried about any differences that you may find, as side to side posture is not as important as front to back posture as a cause of problems, except in the extreme cases of Scoliosis (p.148). There are no specific corrections prescribed for these asymmetries, as your body can cope well, if kept fit and flexible.

Side to side postural asymmetries do not usually change much once you have stopped growing, but they are important in the understanding of the contributing factors to a problem. The exception to this is in the cases where there is a marked difference in the lengths of the legs.

Self-Assessment

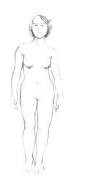

■ Look face on in the mirror and see if one shoulder is higher than the other.

■ Does one side of your pelvis look higher than the other?

■ Are the bony points at the front of your pelvis in the same position on either side?

■ Try standing on something about 0.5–1 cm ($\frac{1}{4}$–$\frac{1}{2}$ in) thick with the shorter leg and see if it makes things look better.

■ If the difference is quite large you may walk with a limp.

Unequal Leg Lengths

Frequently one leg is slightly shorter than the other, which causes the two pelvic bones to twist slightly to compensate for the difference. Your muscles can usually cope with the extra tension, but under stress or fatigue, these muscles are likely to give pain before other muscles that are not working as hard. The asymmetrical position does not cause the symptoms, therefore, but does contribute to their development.

In a typical case the pain will be felt in the low back, buttock and outer thigh muscles of the side of the longer leg. This can be quite severe and is often mistakenly called 'sciatica', in the belief that the pain is due to an irritation of the sciatic nerve.

In these cases the shorter leg can be built up, by wearing pads in your shoes or extra heels. This should be done under the supervision of a qualified therapist.

Sitting Posture

Sitting is one of the activities where poor posture is often in evidence; the choice and design of chairs often makes it impossible to sit without strain for any length of time.

Low Back Area When sitting the low back should not be bent forwards; it should be upright or maintain a slight backwards curve. There are four factors that can help this:

1 **Sitting upright.** Always sit with your sacrum as far back in the seat as you can. Don't slouch.

2 **The Pelvic Tilt** (p.123).

3 **The angle of the seat of the chair.** It helps if it is tilted slightly forwards as this helps to keep your spine upright.

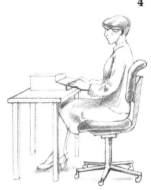

4 **Support in the low back.** The use of chairs with a fairly upright back and good lumbar support helps to prevent strain on the low back. Avoid soft, saggy and unsupporting chairs and car seats. If your chair does not give adequate support, either get another chair or try to make a lumbar support using cushions. Shaped supports that fit into chairs to improve them are available. These are most frequently used in cars, where there are still many seats with very little support. If you do a lot of driving, or already have a low back problem, try to make sure that your back has the support that it needs.

Thoracic and Neck Areas These areas can also be under strain while sitting, especially if you are bending over a desk or drawing board, or are typing. It is important that the height of the chair and desk are adjusted to suit your individual needs, and consideration should be given to the slope of the working surface and the positioning of things that you are looking at. Typists or keyboard operators should take care to avoid always twisting their necks in one direction. Move your work to the other side frequently to minimize the strain.

Even at home you should be careful as many of the soft sofas and armchairs lack upper back and neck support. Many old, straight-backed chairs are more suitable than modern designs.

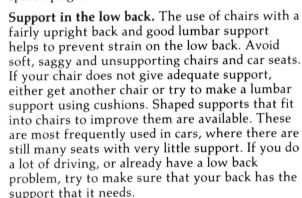

PREVENTION

Other Important Preventative Measures

General Fitness

General fitness involves the mental, emotional and visceral, as well as the physical aspects of an individual. You may think that you are physically fit, but if you are under pressure in any of the other areas you can still be vulnerable to back and neck pain. When considering the prevention of back and neck problems, don't think only about your physical side; think more widely and you will get a more effective, balanced picture. Characteristics necessary for total fitness are:

- Mental and emotional well-being.

- Healthy internal organs.

- Strong muscles to support you and carry out the movements you demand.

- Stamina, so that your body does not tire towards the end of the day.

- Suppleness, to keep your joints and tissues mobile and prevent stiffness.

On the physical side, too great an emphasis is placed on strength at the expense of suppleness and stamina. There are many 'muscle-bound' strongmen who get problems because they do not stretch their tissues, and so lose their elasticity and stiffen up. The Therapeutic Exercises (p.95) will keep you physically fit; Regular Exercise (p.127) will also help you, both mentally and emotionally.

Assess Your Fitness Two simple tests can give a guide to your general fitness and the strength of your heart and lungs. These involve taking your pulse, which is best felt on the underside of your wrist. Count your pulse for fifteen seconds then multiply by four to get the number of beats per minute. The lower your pulse the better.

1 Take your pulse when you are rested and relaxed. Do this first thing in the morning or after the Basic Relaxation Plan (p.79).

2 Take your pulse after doing the following exercise for three minutes: step up and down, moving one foot after the other, onto the lowest of a flight of steps at a rate of approximately twenty four times a minute. Sit down and rest for fifteen seconds, then take your pulse for the next fifteen seconds. Stop the exercise if you feel dizzy or breathless.

	RESTING PULSE RATE		PULSE RECOVERY RATE	
Age	*Men*	*Women*	*Men*	*Women*
20—50	55–85	65–90	70–100	75–110
Over 50	65–90	70–95	80–110	85–115

If your pulse rate in beats per minute is above these figures in either test, you are unfit and should carefully consider your general health. Avoid vigorous exertion until you are fitter. The Mild Routine (p.96), gentle swimming or walking will be safe to start with, then gradually increase your level of exercise over a period of weeks. Make sure you exercise regularly. Do not expect changes immediately as it takes time for your body to adjust.

Regular Exercise

Your body needs regular exercise throughout your life to function well. It should be an automatic process like eating or breathing, but many people unfortunately do little exercise or only exercise spasmodically. A good form of regular exercise will help unwind tension and aid your breathing, digestion and circulation.

The form of exercise that suits you depends on your individual needs, lifestyle, physique and motivation, but an exercise, or routine, should ideally be:

■ **Enjoyable.** You should be able to relax and leave your tensions behind when doing it, and you should feel good afterwards.

■ **Complete.** It should exercise your whole body.

■ **Safe.** It should not damage any part of your body. Beware of over-exercising which can cause your muscles to fatigue and be sore, and leave you vulnerable to injury.

■ **Convenient.** It should fit into and become part of your lifestyle; you will not be able to keep it up for years unless this is so.

Your exercise can therefore be divided into three categories:

1 **Normal everyday activity.** If you lead an active life, you will probably need to do less additional exercise than someone who is mainly sedentary. Everyday activity, however, is not usually totally sufficient, as it doesn't always exercise the whole body, tending not to include much stretching or relaxing. It also fails to exercise the muscles that really need it, because it reinforces the postural faults that you already have.

2 **Sport.** This activity usually involves the coordinated use of much of the body. The best 'all-rounder' is swimming, particularly if you have a back problem, as the water supports you and your weight is not transmitted through your spine. Swimming can also be done at any age.

3 **Exercise Routines.** These can vary from ten minutes exercise at home to a supervised gym workout or stretch class. Yoga, keep-fit and Tai Chi are other examples. Provided that they satisfy the basic criteria outlined above, these can all be very good for you. Make sure that you have an experienced supervisor or teacher when you do these exercises, especially if you are a beginner.

Do a variety of sports or routines and keep up some sort of exercise regularly; your muscles and other tissues stiffen up and weaken very quickly. Two weeks between sessions is too long.

Age should not stop you from exercising. When you are older, however, you should use less force and exertion and not expect to be quite as supple as you were before. It is just as important that you keep active when you are ninety as it was when you were twenty.

Maintaining Back Fitness

It is impossible to devise a programme that will suit everyone; your own routine should fit in with your own and your family's life. You should plan to do something everyday, however, no matter how little. A typical week might go something like this:

Monday. Mild Routine (p.96) and Basic Relaxation Plan (p.79).

Tuesday. Intermediate Routine (p.102).

Wednesday. Swimming.

Thursday. Mild Routine and Basic Relaxation Plan.

Friday. Dancing, or a yoga class.

Saturday. Sport, swimming, gym workout or the Vigorous Routine (p.105).

Sunday. Basic Relaxation Plan, perhaps followed by a brisk walk.

This list gives an idea of the sort of things you should think about. Most of the suggestions are not time-consuming – less than half an hour a day on average.

If you prefer, get your family and friends to join in, although it can sometimes be good to have time to yourself. A busy mother can ask her husband to look after the children for half an hour, while she goes to a quiet room to stretch and relax. An over-worked executive can go for a swim in his lunch hour, and do the Basic Relaxation Plan (p.79) after supper. If you are unemployed keep your spirits up by working out in a gym or at home during the day.

Have a good think and plan what you intend to do, without being overambitious. Make sure you stick to your plan, especially if you don't feel like doing it, as that is the time when you are likely to benefit from it the most. Remember, no-one can force you to get fit, so the motivation is up to you and how highly you rate your health.

If you follow the advice given in the rest of this chapter, you should be fit and healthy and feel good. Your spine is perfectly capable of supporting you for your whole life if you treat it, and yourself, well. So be optimistic and get out there and do it – you can if you want to.

PREVENTION

Lifting

The low back is most vulnerable while lifting. Problems frequently occur in this area among heavy manual workers, and in professions, such as nursing, where a lot of lifting is done.

There are several points to note if you wish to minimize the strain of lifting:

- Do not try to lift anything that is too heavy for you. If something is heavy, separate it into smaller loads, for instance, by partially unloading a box, or get someone to help you.

- Stand with your feet apart and bend your knees, keeping your spine relatively upright. Use your leg muscles to provide the power rather than your back muscles. Avoid bending forwards to lift anything.

- Keep the load as close to your body as possible. Grip the load firmly and make sure that it is well balanced.

- Do not twist your spine while lifting; keep yourself well balanced and move your feet to turn your whole body, rather than twisting your back.

- Use the Pelvic Tilt (p.123) while lifting, as this makes sure that your stomach muscles take some of the load. Good tone and strength in your stomach muscles is essential if you lift frequently as they support and strengthen the low back.

Correct Lifting

The figure on the left shows how not to lift, as bending forwards puts a great strain on your spine. The figure on the right is lifting correctly, with bent knees and straight spine. In this way the leg and stomach muscles take some of the strain off the back muscles.

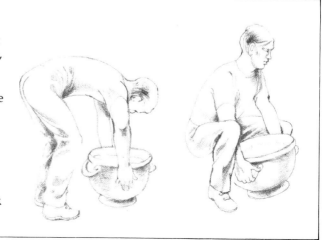

- If carrying loads by your side, such as suitcases or shopping, try to distribute the load evenly. If this is impractical, swap the load from side to side frequently and have rests if necessary.

- If you have a choice, pull rather than push a load, as there is more pressure on the low back when pushing.

- Avoid heavy lifting when you are tired or ill, as your muscles will be weaker and less able to protect you. Do not lift anything at all if you are recovering from a disc herniation in the low back.

- Plan your movements to minimize the amount of bending and lifting that you have to do. Correct heights for work surfaces and the use of labour-saving devices, such as ovens mounted higher on the wall, are useful to minimize strain.

Sleeping

Beds Most people with healthy spines are able to cope with all sorts of sleeping surfaces, from the floor to old, very soft, spring beds. However, the sleeping surface is important, both from a healing and preventative point of view.

The surface needs enough give to be comfortable, but enough firmness to support your spine along its whole length without allowing it to sag. Usually this is achieved by

Mattresses and Pillows

A sagging mattress (above) can put strain on the lumbar spine. A firm, but comfortable mattress (below) supports the spine along its whole length. It is important to sleep with the correct pillow width; the spine should be straight from head to pelvis.

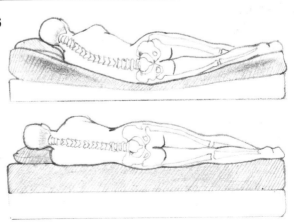

having a solid base, such as slatted pine, and a well-made firm mattress on top or, if preferred, a thick futon. While asleep we change our position many times, and this is easier to do on a firm rather than a sagging mattress.

Putting the mattress on the floor is only a good idea in an emergency, as getting up and down from a low bed can be difficult; a board under the mattress is better if you urgently need a firmer surface. Be wary of expensive orthopaedic beds: good support can be found at reasonable cost.

Pillows   When you lie on your side you need a pillow that is the width of one shoulder to fill the gap between your head and the bed, without letting your head drop down or pushing it up. When you lie on your back you need only a thin pillow or none at all. The pillow required therefore depends on your size and sleeping position. Some pillows, such as feather, can be bunched up or flattened to alter their height, and there are pillows designed to be thinner in the middle than at the ends, to accommodate changes of position.

Position   The principal benefit of lying down is that your weight is not transmitted through your spine as it is when you are standing or sitting. Any position of lying down accomplishes this, but lying on your back or sides is better than lying face down, as in this position you can't bend your knees up and it can strain the neck.

Getting out of Bed

Keep your spine straight while getting out of bed by turning onto your side and bending your knees up together. Drop your lower legs over the side of the bed; use their weight to raise your torso, and at the same time push yourself up with your arms. Try to do this in one smooth movement. Reverse the sequence when lying down.

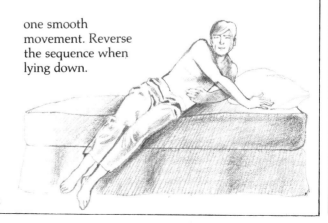

Getting out of bed You are vulnerable in the first few minutes of the day, as your discs are thick and your muscular co-ordination a little poor. A quick stretch and a few exercises before getting up (see Mild Routine p.96) is a good idea, and getting out of the bed in a way that avoids twisting helps. This is particularly important if you are suffering from a low back problem, such as disc herniation.

Relaxation Being asleep does not mean that you are relaxed; your subconscious, which controls the patterns of tension in your body, is very active. This can be seen in the number of people who grind their teeth, or are restless, during sleep. If a pattern of tension is anything more than transitory, it will be the same when you wake up as when you went to sleep. You should consult the section on Relaxation (p.79).

Sex This is possible with most back problems though your partner will have to do most of the work. If you have a disc herniation, nerve irritation or a sacro-iliac ligament problem, lie on your back or side and do not move too much. Muscular tension or spasm may be eased once your muscles have warmed up, so experiment; you may find that you can be active without causing pain or even end up with less pain.

Nutrition

There are many claims for various diets and supplements and while some of them may benefit some people, most should be thought about critically.

There are a few situations where nutrition is important in relation to physical (and mental) problems; most of these can be helped by following a low-stress diet, which as the name implies, is not too much for your body to cope with and gives it good nutrients. This is also a good diet to follow if you are suffering from stress or recovering from illness.

Low-Stress Diet Avoid or reduce sugar, white flour, any refined or processed foods, additives such as colourings, flavourings and preservatives, alcohol, salt, coffee, cola and chocolate.

PREVENTION

- Eat plenty of fresh vegetables (especially raw), salads, fish, fresh fruit, whole-grain cereals, beans, brown rice, yoghurt (made with goat's milk, if you have food allergies) and free-range chicken.

- Do not fry your food, and use only good vegetable oils and margarines rather than lard or butter.

- Eat your meals regularly three times a day, even if your appetite is poor; make sure especially that you have a good breakfast, as missing it can cause a low blood sugar level later in the morning.

- Eat slowly and chew your food well.

- Vitamin C is the only supplement that most people seem to need, especially if they are ill, under stress or smoke. This can be obtained from citrus fruits and juices, or as a tablet. A daily dose of 250 mg should be sufficient.

Arthritis Rheumatoid arthritis is a condition that affects all the tissues of the body, not just the joints. Generally people feel better in the long-term if they follow the low-stress diet and consider the possibility of food intolerances or allergies.

Osteoporosis This is a condition where your bones become thinner and weaker in old age. Occasionally this happens earlier, especially in a percentage of post-menopausal women, due to the hormonal changes. You may find that taking the following supplements helps in the long term:

- Calcium, which is found in dairy products and cereals, or taken as tablets.

- Vitamin D, which sunlight encourages your skin to produce. Get into the sunshine as often as you can; if you cannot , take cod liver oil every day.

- Take regular exercise as this also helps to keep the bones strong.

Nerve Symptoms There is evidence to suggest that B vitamins, especially B1 and B12, can help to improve the function of nerves. It is best to take a good multiple B-complex supplement rather than individual vitamins.

Migraine Various foods and chemicals can trigger migraine in susceptible individuals. Sufferers may benefit from trying the following exclusion diet for a month, and then adding the foods back again to see if there is any reaction. Follow the low-stress diet and avoid yeast extracts and products, cheese, sausages, salami, oranges, wheat, cow's milk, smoking and the contraceptive pill.

Protein Deficiency Weakness of muscles and consequent overtightening and pain occasionally occurs in people who don't eat enough protein. Most vulnerable to this are people who are very faddish about food, such as some vegans, or people who rush around and miss meals. If your muscles look thin and weak and your diet is poor, then eat more protein; fish is probably the best source.

Allergies Many reactions called 'allergic' are not true allergies, but are food intolerances – chemical reactions to chemicals in the food. An example of this is coffee, which affects a lot of people, as it contains many powerful chemicals; this reaction is not a true allergy. True allergy is an inherited characteristic and is associated with asthma, eczema, hay fever and dust reactions.

Major allergens in your diet should be avoided; the best test is to eliminate the suspect food from your diet for a few weeks, then eat it again and see how you feel. Try not to become obsessed, as allergies are associated with stress and the more worried you become the more allergies you will create. Look at other areas of your life and try to understand what may be making your system over-sensitive. Take steps to change, or adjust, them rather than blaming your food.

Breathing

Breathing is one of the necessary functions of the body that most people could do in a more relaxed and efficient manner. This will help to prevent many back and neck problems from occurring. Correct breathing aids the circulation and the movement of organs and tissues throughout the whole of your torso.

There are three main points to remember:

1 Normal quiet breathing should be done using the diaphragm and abdominal muscles. Many people do not do this and in the long-term many of their body functions can suffer, especially the circulation and the mobility of the digestive tract.

2 The ribs and upper chest should only be used when taking a deep breath or when breathing hard during exertion. Too often people use their ribs all the time which can make the muscles that control them very tired and tight.

3 Breathing out is just as important as breathing in. Many states of tension and anxiety cause you to hold your breath; in the long-term the muscles that produce this movement, particularly those in the upper back, neck and between the ribs, become tight and shortened, so that breathing out becomes difficult. This anxious upper chest breathing pattern can also be part of 'hyperventilation', which can lead to pins and needles, dizziness and feelings of insecurity.

Test and Improve Your Breathing Put both hands on your abdomen and breathe in and out slowly; try to push your hand out with your stomach as you breathe in and let your hand go in as

Learning to Breathe Using Your Abdominal Muscles

Lie on your back in a comfortable position and put your hands on your stomach so that you can feel the muscles move as you breathe. Imagine that there is a balloon inside your stomach that fills with air and expands in all directions as you breathe in, and then slowly deflates as you breathe out. Your upper ribs and chest should stay relaxed while doing this.

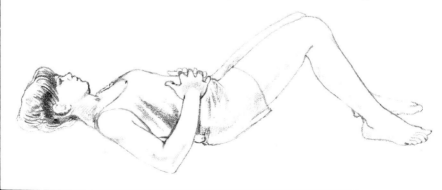

you breathe out. You may find this difficult if you are not used to it but practice will help. It can be done while you are lying, sitting or standing. If you have a large overweight abdomen or weak or flabby abdominal muscles you may need to lose weight and exercise your muscles. If you learn to breathe using your abdominal muscles it will help to keep them in trim.

If your shoulders and upper ribs are held upwards, let them down and gently breathe out more with your upper ribs with each breath that you take. If you have had chronic tension in the area you may need to massage the muscles in the front and back of your chest and neck to help them relax.

Make your cycle of breathing even, so that you breathe out for the same length of time as you breathe in. Make sure that you are not in the habit of holding your breath.

Gradually, if you breathe slowly and deeply you may start to feel more integrated and whole within your body. Each breath will feel as if it is filling your abdomen, and even moving your pelvis and low back. This is a good state to achieve, as it is not only relaxing but also helps to improve and maintain the strength, coordination and mobility of many of your body's tissues.

Warmth

Muscles are the most important tissues in the body in relation to its functioning and correct movement. They are also the source of most aches and pains. Muscles hurt when they are contracted, as the blood flow through them is reduced. Cold temperatures and draughts reduce the blood flow further and make your muscles contract to try and keep you warm. Thus keeping warm is essential to prevent the general state of tension in your muscles from building up, which makes you vulnerable to back and neck pains.

If the cold is just on a local area of the body the muscles there can get very tense and painful after a while. The areas most often affected are the neck, especially when sitting by an open window with a draught, and the low back, when bending forwards and leaving a gap between your shirt and trousers. Treatment is as for Muscular Tension (p.39).

Risk Factors to Avoid

There are certain factors in your daily life which may put you specially at risk from back and neck pain. This chapter concentrates on four areas of your life where you can take active steps to minimize your chances of either suffering back and neck pain or of aggravating your problem further.

Excess Weight

The most frequent problems associated with incorrect weight are due to overweight, though some people are underweight because of illness or anorexia, which causes their muscles to become weak and tight. Being heavier for your height, sex and build is one of the most common problems in the western world and contributes to many problems, from heart failure to diabetes and musculo-skeletal strains.

One of the main functions of your back is to support you; the heavier you are the more work the back has to do to achieve this. Frequently the bulk of the excess weight is carried in the front of the stomach area. This places additional strain on the low back, as it pulls you forwards, making your muscles work hard to keep you upright. Overweight people also tend to do less exercise, so their muscles, especially at the front and sides of the trunk, tend to be in poor condition.

Overweight is not just associated with muscle problems but is also a major contributing factor to the development of disc herniation and degenerative changes (not only in the spine but also in the legs).

Self-Help If you know your weight is really excessive (normally your body can tolerate a little extra without any trouble), you have to lose it for your long-term health and fitness.

The first step in losing weight is to ask yourself whether or not, deep down, you really want to lose weight. A lot of people feel they need to be overweight for a variety of reasons, such as insecurity and the need to have a cushion against the world, or the need to appear big and strong physically. Often the inability to lose weight, or keep it off once you have lost it, is because of these deeper tensions and stresses which you may not consciously be aware of.

Think about your current circumstances and also times earlier in your life, perhaps when you first became overweight, and try to answer the question 'Why do I need to be heavy?' Sorting out these deeper motives is complicated, but the more you understand about yourself, the more likely you are to feel comfortable and secure at a lower weight.

Occasionally hormonal and metabolic problems can cause weight gain, but this is usually just an excuse, as hormones can change as your body and emotions change.

The practical remedies are principally diet and exercise. You need to do both to lose weight successfully, as the exercise not only burns up the fat stores but also, in the long-term, raises your metabolic rate so the fat is less likely to return.

Your diet can be one of the many available plans or slimming aids. Beware of any artificial substitute meals out of a packet, as they can upset your digestion and, despite their claims, are unlikely to be as beneficial as good food.

Eat plenty of salads and vegetables, and a reasonable amount of fruit. For protein eat fish or beans. Whole grains such as brown rice or muesli are acceptable in limited amounts, the latter eaten with soya milk. Avoid any fatty things, such as dairy products (especially butter), meat, oils and sauces. Also avoid sugary or starchy foods, such as sweets, cakes, biscuits and bread. If you need a snack between meals eat some carrots or an apple.

For exercise do whatever you enjoy doing. Swimming and walking are good, as are many of the modern gyms with specially designed equipment. Try to exercise every day in a way that makes you feel as if you have done something (see Regular Exercise p.127). Lastly, remember that losing weight can be quite a stressful process, so take your mind off things and spoil yourself a bit: visit people or places that you enjoy, have massages, go to the cinema or paint a picture. Then the changes will occur more easily.

Occupational Hazards

What you do for many hours each week is often an important factor in the production of back and neck problems. You should think about what you do and to consider ways in which you can minimize the physical and mental stresses involved.

Sedentary or Desk Jobs The crucial factors here are the strains from sitting (see Sitting Posture p.125), the lack of exercise, and the tension that can be generated without being able to burn it off physically. Get into the habit of moving about, stretching your neck and shoulders at the desk (see Sitting Routine p.112), and briskly walking to and from work and in your lunch break. If convenient go to a gym or have a swim several times a week. Try to take up a sport or hobby that involves exercise you can do regularly at weekends.

Computer screens, fluorescent lights, air-conditioning, poor ventilation and smoky atmospheres can all contribute to stress and tension and lead to fatigue and inefficiency in the working environment.

Lifting and Bending Building work, carpet laying and gardening are potentially damaging occupations, particularly for your low back. Avoid incorrect Lifting (p.130) and prolonged bending by the correct positioning of work surfaces, kneeling or using aids (such as long handled tools for gardeners). If you really cannot avoid bending, you must keep the muscles round your trunk in good tone and avoid Excess Weight (p.139) as this adds to the strain.

Driving This can be a strain on the low back because of the Sitting Posture (p.125), and a strain on the neck and shoulders because of the concentration involved and the use of the arms. Test the seats when choosing a car to make sure that you are supported and the seats can be adjusted to suit other drivers. If you find that there is inadequate lumbar support, buy a patent device to remedy this. Try to relax your neck and shoulders while you are driving and don't grip the steering wheel too tightly. If you are driving a long distance stop regularly and walk about and stretch. Do the Sitting Routine (p.112) regularly.

Housework, Cleaning and Shopping These and other occupations which involve standing all day have their own potential stresses. If there is anything that you do that hurts your back or neck, or feels uncomfortable, work out a way of doing it with less strain. For example, if you are standing all day try to keep moving, by standing on tip-toes, bending your knees and tensing and relaxing different groups of muscles, such as your thighs, stomach and buttocks; in other words keep active. If you are shopping, don't try to carry too much. Get a trolley or basket on wheels. If you are in pain lie down and do the Basic Relaxation Plan (p.79) when you have a chance.

Sports Stresses

Sports are, on the whole, a good way of exercising and keeping fit, however they are not without their potential dangers in terms of causing or aggravating problems. Many problems associated with sport occur in the limbs either through overuse, such as tennis elbow, or twists and falls, such as a pulled knee or ankle ligament. These are outside the scope of this book.

In terms of the prevention of back and neck problems as a result of sport there are several precautions to take:

■ Do not overdo it. Do not try to do too much too soon, or play when you are fatigued or ill. You are most vulnerable when you are starting a sport for the first time or taking it up again after a time. Start gently, well within your capabilities and gradually build up to a full game, whatever the sport, over one to three months – depending on your fitness.

■ Learn to play the sport properly, and get good equipment if necessary. For instance, if you start road running or jogging, get good shoes with shock absorbing soles to prevent jarring of your legs and back. If starting a sport like golf, have lessons so that you get your swing right and prevent backstrain due to a bad swing.

■ Listen to your body, rest if your back hurts and treat it if it persists or recurs. Swimming is usually safe for most back problems, so if in doubt do this in as relaxed a manner as you can, with a variety of strokes, and if you feel confident do some gentle stretching exercises in the water.

Disc Herniation All sport should be avoided until you are well recovered. Unfortunately discs are a bit vulnerable for up to eighteen months after the symptoms have eased so care should be taken. The best sport at this time is swimming.

Sacro-Iliac Ligament Problems Avoid twisting movements, such as golf, squash and tennis, until it is settled down. Consider wearing a support belt, and look at your posture and the way you play the sport to see if you are putting strain on one side of your pelvis.

Muscular Spasm and Acute Joint Locking Whether this is in the neck or low back areas, you should avoid sport until the acute phase has subsided, which is usually within two or three days, then relax, warm up and exercise as usual.

Muscular Tension This should actually be eased by most sports once you have warmed up. It is a good idea to relax and warm up first by doing the Mild Routine (p.96). You may feel stiff after the game or the next morning, in which case Massage (p.82) to ease tight fibres in the muscles is recommended.

Stress

Stress is the term used to describe the results of strains, imbalances and changes, within and outside you. These can result from physical, mental, nutritional or environmental influences.

Mental and emotional stresses such as financial worries and relationship problems, chemical stresses such as eating 'junk food', and physical stresses such as overwork will make you vulnerable and more likely to develop back and neck pain. However it is not only negative influences that can cause stress; positive events, such as moving house, marriage and even going on holiday can be stressful too. Most major changes in your life are stressful to some extent.

In a mild degree stress can be stimulating, but it can rapidly accumulate and overwhelm you. Every person reacts differently to differing situations and each individual has a different ability to cope with stress and a different threshold, above which symptoms will develop. There is also a time factor involved; if stress is spread out over a long period, you may cope with it more easily. Once a stressful event has occurred, it can take time to recover.

Symptoms The ways in which symptoms of stress manifest themselves depends on the individual. Some of the areas that can change are:

- **Hormones and metabolism.** Overproduction of adrenaline causes sweating, rapid pulse and high blood pressure.

- **Muscles.** These get tense, which may result in headaches, shaking and high blood pressure.

- **Mind.** Your sleep patterns may alter and you can suffer from lethargy, depression, poor concentration and panic.

If the stress is prolonged, these can cause permanent changes. High blood pressure can strain the heart and chronic muscular tension in the back or neck can affect your posture.

Avoiding Stress Some major stresses are difficult to alter consciously as their main effects are subconscious. You may consciously think that you have not been affected by an event, when in reality the undercurrent of tension can cause a variety of problems. Family problems and relationship difficulties are often underestimated in this way. If you start to get any warning signs of stress, look at the ways you can deal with it:

- **Physical stress.** Rest (p.78), Relaxation (p.79) and Regular Exercise (p.127); pace yourself so that you are not doing too much at once.

- **Emotional stress.** Communicate and show your feelings to others. Forget events that have upset you or gone wrong in the past.

- **Metabolic stress.** Eat well and regularly for good Nutrition (page 133).

- **Mental stress.** Relaxation (p.79), breathe deeply and get things in perspective. Establish realistic goals to aim for, to give yourself both motivation and the satisfaction of achievement.

Nobody can avoid stress totally; to try to do so would in itself be a stressful obsession. However, you can reduce its worst effects by an awareness of the pace of life that suits you. Ultimately this may involve a change in your lifestyle, responsibilities and attitudes.

Special Conditions

*T*his chapter covers some specific spinal problems that were referred to in previous chapters, but not dealt with fully. It is not exhaustive, however, and the details are necessarily limited. It also explains some general situations that might have an effect on the health of your spine and which you may wish to know more about.

Spinal Conditions

Arthritis

This literally means inflammation of a joint, although it is also used to describe degenerative changes. The three most prevalent types of arthritis are described in this section; details of other types, such as gout, infective arthritis and the arthritis of rheumatic fever, may be found in a medical textbook.

Osteoarthritis This is a degenerative process caused by the wear and tear of a joint. It tends to occur naturally with age and is most found in the joints under the greatest load, thus mainly the spine and lower limbs. It is increased if there has been previous damage or disease of the joint, and is more likely if you are overweight. In the spine the process is called spondylarthrosis, and the areas that show most changes are usually the base of the spine, the thoracic area and the base of the neck.

Osteoarthritis is a gradual process and usually causes no symptoms other than stiffness; the cartilage, which covers the bones, wears first and is not sensitive to pain. In the rarer advanced cases, the discomfort can be severe.

Rheumatoid Arthritis This is a chronic inflammatory condition which can start at any age and affect several joints, particularly the hands, wrists, feet, knees and elbows. The spine is not usually badly affected, although the top of the neck is sometimes vulnerable. It is associated with inflammatory conditions throughout the body and can be regarded as a generalized illness, rather than just a joint condition. The cause is largely unknown, although genetic factors and stress play a part.

There are several approaches to treatment depending on severity. In some cases diet changes seem to help (see Nutrition p.133), and most therapies claim to be of benefit. It is not an easy condition to treat and medical opinion should be sought in any case. It tends to burn itself out after months or years, sometimes leaving the affected joints damaged.

SPECIAL CONDITIONS

Ankylosing Spondylitis

This is principally a disease of the spine, consisting of an inflammation, which then progresses to bony ankylosis (fusion) of the affected spinal segments. It begins in the sacro-iliac joints and travels up the spine, often reaching as far as the neck.

The causes of ankylosing spondylitis are unknown, although there is evidence that it is partly hereditary. It generally only affects men, beginning between the ages of eighteen and thirty and usually burning itself out after several years. Blood tests can confirm it in an active phase and medical opinion should be sought in any case.

Osteochondritis

This is a process that affects a large percentage of people to some degree. During the teenage years, the bodies of one or more vertebrae become temporarily softer and wedge-shaped, which results in thinning of the adjacent discs. Osteochondritis is usually painless and occurs without you being aware of it, although the changes can be seen on X-ray plates. Occasionally it is painful and can affect a number of vertebrae; this is called active osteochondritis, which can last up to two years.

The final effects are a vertebra, or group of vertebrae, which is very stiff and bent forwards in a wedge shape. This in itself causes no symptoms, but it does put more strain on adjacent vertebrae, as they have to compensate for the lack of mobility.

As the process usually occurs in the thoracic spine, which is fairly stiff and curved forwards anyway, it has little effect. Osteochondritis causes more problems when it occurs in the upper lumbar spine, or the junction of the lumbar and thoracic spines, as these areas should move freely and be curved backwards. The stiffness and wedging that result put strain on the lower lumbar spine making it more vulnerable to injury and strain.

Osteochondritis is usually no problem in itself, but can be a major contributing factor to the development of problems in unaffected areas. Once it has occurred it cannot be reversed, although keeping the affected area as mobile as possible is beneficial.

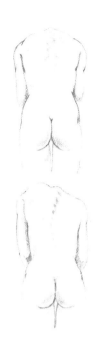

Scoliosis

This means a curvature of the spine in a lateral, or side to side, direction (see Side to Side Posture p.123). You may develop a temporary scoliosis due to muscle spasm caused by acute low back pain. This is there to protect you and stop further damage if, for example, a disc or a nerve is involved; it will go when the spasm eases.

True scoliosis, which is structural and permanent, occasionally develops in childhood or adolescence. This can be relatively minor, often passing unnoticed, or it can be more major and cause great deformity. The cause of severe scolioses is sometimes a malformed vertebra, but is often unknown. Treatment depends on severity and the opinion of an orthopaedic specialist should be sought. The twisted bones are not painful, but the muscles that keep you upright have to work harder; pain in these can be treated as for Muscular Tension (p.56).

Spondylolisthesis

This means the displacement of a vertebra forwards upon the vertebra below it. It usually occurs in the lumbar spine and is generally caused by a maldevelopment of the pillars of bone that normally prevent this displacement from happening. There is evidence that it can be caused by injury or stress fractures. The displacement is usually of a small degree, though occasionally it does progress further, particularly in growing children, and threatens to compress the nerves at the base of the spine, in which case surgery may be necessary to stabilize it.

Many cases of this give no symptoms and are only picked up by chance on an X-ray. Sometimes symptoms do occur due to the strain put on the adjacent structures, such as the disc, ligaments and muscles, by the dispacement.

Treatment is aimed at stabilizing the displacement and easing the strain on the surrounding tissues. Postural changes are important to keep the lumbar spine relatively straight and minimize further displacement; the Pelvic Tilt (p.123) is particularly effective.

Other Conditions

Aging

Once your spine has finished growing in your early twenties, it gradually begins to show the changes that occur naturally with time. These happen at different rates in different individuals, and can include a loss of flexibility, poorer circulation and slower healing. In the spine the process is called 'spondylosis' and the most obvious changes occur in the discs, beginning with the gradual loss of fluidity of the central nucleus and small tears appearing in the annulus. As a result the discs become thinner, causing:

■ a shortening of the spine of up to 2 cm (1 in);

■ a reduction in the range of movement allowed by the discs, which combined with the loss of elasticity, makes the spine stiffer;

■ an alternation in the stresses put on the facet joints, so that they show signs of wear and tear, such as worn joint surfaces (see Arthritis p.146);

■ changes in the bone of the vertebrae with the formation of osteophytes, which are usually no trouble, although they occasionally irritate nerves, especially in the neck.

Degenerative Changes

As you get older your spine naturally undergoes some degenerative changes: the discs become thinner and less flexible; the cartilage in the joints becomes worn, possibly causing arthritis; the vertebrae thicken to form projections of bone, called osteophytes, which can irritate nearby nerves (right).

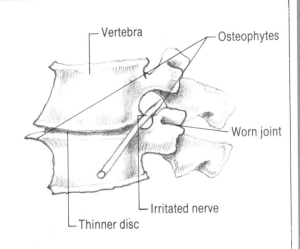

Vertebra

Osteophytes

Worn joint

Irritated nerve

Thinner disc

In old age, or after the menopause in women, the bones can also become weaker due to a loss of minerals, making them more brittle and vulnerable to fracture. This process is called osteoporosis and diet may help to reduce its severity (see Nutrition p.133).

These sound like unpleasant changes, but they are part of the natural aging process and you shouldn't panic or be worried that you have some terrible disease; your bones are constantly changing throughout your life, making new bone and destroying old.

Pain is not a normal feature of aging; if you are suffering, you should do something about it, rather than 'having to live with it', as older people are often told (see Degenerative Changes p.48).

Self-Help These changes occur gradually over many years, so the first step is to prevent excessive strain on your spine throughout your life by:

- making sure that you lose any Excess Weight (p.139).

- keeping fit and mobile with Regular Exercise (p.127).

- attention to Posture (p.121).

Over the age of fifty the above are still important, especially keeping active and mobile. Many people keep active with walking and perhaps a gentle routine of exercise well into their eighties and beyond. Nutrition (p.133), should be considered, as should self-help measures such as Relaxation (p.79).

One bit of good news is that severe acute back and neck pains and disc herniations are rare over fifty even if you had them in your earlier years.

Childhood

Back and neck problems are uncommon in children. The only major ones that occur are Scoliosis (p.148), Spondylolisthesis (p.148) and some rare developmental anomalies. If you wish to test for scoliosis, have the child stripped to the waist facing away from you. Look for asymmetries in the shape of the spine, height of the shoulders and curvature of the hips. Ask the child to bend forwards away from you; if you can see an obvious asymmetrical lump it may be due to a structural scoliosis.

Posture is very important, although this varies and changes a great deal in toddlers and infants and you shouldn't worry too much about it, however unusual it looks. If after the age of eight the child's posture seems bad, work out the causes by referring to Posture (p.121).

If it is due to copying poor parental posture, the parents should consider improving theirs! If it is a result of weak muscles caused by illness, encourage regular exercise to regain fitness and stamina; swimming is particularly good. If it is a result of emotional tensions, do your best to understand and resolve the pressures on the child; consider seeing a family therapist.

If the posture remains poor, encourage the child to visit a therapist who specializes in postural problems, such as a teacher of the Alexander Technique. It is important that good posture should be established before the late teens, as this is when the spine stops growing and changes become more difficult to achieve. You should bear in mind, however, that lasting improvements take several months to achieve.

Pain in the back or neck is unusual in children, so if a child complains of these symptoms, it is advisable to consult a qualified therapist.

Illness

Illness is important in back and neck pain, as your muscles have less stamina and are more likely to get tense. Many illnesses, especially viruses, also directly cause aches in muscles and joints. There are two questions to ask if you are ill:

How did I become ill? Often the answer to this is long and complex, perhaps including family or childhood vulnerabilities, such as a weak chest in an asthmatic. Usually some more immediate factors also contribute, such as fatigue or worry. The more you understand your illness and how you react to it, the easier it is to resolve it, and perhaps prevent it from happening again.

What is stopping me from being healthy?

Obstacles to health are often found in many different areas from your body to diet, emotional stresses and hostile environment. Identify the most immediate obstacle and work on it; when that is overcome work on the next and so on.

Becoming ill often takes a long time, as does getting better. You may think that you are better before you really are, causing you to relapse or never totally recover. If you need some help in understanding your illness and becoming healthy, don't be afraid to seek it, whoever you consult. There are many views on health and ill-health, so if one approach does not suit you try another.

Pregnancy

Pregnancy is generally a very healthy time and many conditions get better as the body changes. Unfortunately low back pain occurs fairly often during pregnancy for two reasons:

1   The weight of the growing baby and enlarged fluid-filled uterus tends to pull you forwards, so the muscles in your low back and buttocks have to work harder to hold you up. The muscles in the upper back also take more strain as your breasts get larger and heavier. Your posture will change to compensate, but your spine needs to be flexible.

2   The changes in your hormones cause the ligaments around the sacro-iliac joints to soften and the joints to become more mobile, which aids labour. This means that the sacro-iliac ligaments are more prone to becoming overstretched and inflamed.

The strain on the lower back can be prevented by making sure your centre of gravity does not fall too far forwards. Tip your pelvis backwards using the Pelvic Tilt (p.123) and keep your spine feeling long. Keeping your muscles in good condition can prevent them from hurting. Exercise can be continued right through pregnancy and there are now many classes specifically catering for the needs of pregnant women. You can do exercises yourself, particularly the Mild Routine (p.96).

Correct Posture During Pregnancy

The increase in weight at the front of the body during pregnancy places a strain on the spine, which can be reduced by attention to posture. The figure on the left shows the posture often assumed during pregnancy, with the lumbar spine excessively curved inwards to compensate for the additional weight. The figure on the right shows the improved posture that can be achieved by practising the Pelvic Tilt and the Neck Lengthening exercises.

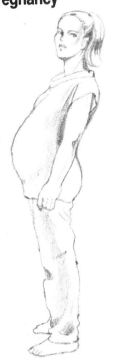
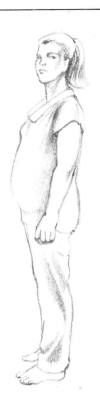

If the sacro-iliac ligaments are inflamed, it is best to let the inflammation calm down by avoiding strain on the back. You may find that lying on your back is uncomfortable in the later stages of pregnancy, and can cause the rare examples of genuine sacro-iliac locking, in which case lie on your side.

If the pain is persistent consult a qualified therapist. There is no evidence that gentle massage or manipulative treatment can cause a miscarriage. In most cases the symptoms ease once the baby has been born and your strength is recovered.

During labour any back pain can often be eased by moving about, warmth on the back muscles from a hot water bottle, or by gentle massage from your partner. Even just having a hand supporting your back can be very comforting. After delivery your muscles will gradually recover their tone. When you feel strong enough, exercises are very useful, particularly to tighten up your abdominal muscles and give your back full support. The Mild Routine (p.96) is safe and effective if done daily.

Breastfeeding and carrying the baby can be a strain on the muscles in the upper back so try to help them by gentle massage and heat. Take care when lifting your children as they get bigger and heavier!

Visceral Problems

The viscera are your internal systems, such as the heart, lungs and kidneys. Problems with these organs can affect your spine. Many visceral problems, such as a chest infection, are reasonably easy to diagnose; sometimes, however, it is less easy to distinguish visceral from musculo-skeletal problems, even for trained practitioners.

Severe visceral problems are best dealt with quickly by your doctor or hospital. The more chronic, less immediately threatening, visceral problems can be treated in a number of ways. Some of the methods outlined in this book can help to improve visceral function. For example, many chest problems can be helped by improving the mobility of the thoracic area and relaxing the muscles, and some digestive and pelvic problems can be eased by relaxing the low back and pelvis. Good health and fitness involves all aspects of your life; these aspects are interdependent, so improvements in one area will help problems in the others.

General Diagnostic Features

If pain is the major symptom the key is to work out what affects the pain. Take as an example pain in the front or sides of the chest. Many people immediately think it is their heart and panic: don't. Turn your spine from side to side, take deep breaths in and out and feel around the area with your fingers.

If it is worse with movement or stretching, or the muscles feel contracted and tender, it is likely to be the muscles and ribs that are the problem.

Fever, weakness, sweating, nausea,

breathlessness, or blood in the urine, mean that your problem is mainly visceral and you should see your doctor. If you are in any doubt you should consult your doctor.

Low Back Area Pain

Menstrual pains can be felt in the low back, usually as a diffuse ache in the centre and perhaps spreading to both sides. Some relief may be gained by relaxing the pelvis and low back by better Breathing (p.135). This is also a possible preventative treatment in the long term.

Kidney problems, particularly infections, can cause a deep, usually one-sided, ache in the area between the low back and thoracic areas, spreading down into the front of the pelvis. Such a condition would be associated with symptoms such as fever, malaise and discoloured urine.

Piles can cause coccyx pain, which can lead to muscular tension in the low back and buttocks.

Thoracic Area Pain

Lung problems, especially pleurisy, can cause pain in the chest, often round the side. This is generally associated with symptoms of a chest infection, such as fever, breathlessness, productive cough and malaise.

Heart problems, such as angina or a heart attack, cause severe chest pains. These are associated with pain down the inside of the left or both arms. Usually there will also be shock, breathlessness, weakness or even collapse with such an incident. This is a medical emergency and treatment should be sought at once, unless it is a recurring angina and you are already under medical supervision.

Neck Area Pain

Meningitis, caused by an inflammation or infection of the membranes surrounding the brain and spinal cord, can cause pain and rigidity in the neck. This is usually associated with headache, fever, weakness, nausea and, if allowed to progress, loss of consciousness.

Tonsillitis, or other chronic throat infections, can cause weakness and pain in the muscles in the front of the neck. This in turn can upset the relative balance of the muscles of the neck and contribute to pain in the muscles at the back of the neck, and a tension headache. This can persist even after the throat infection has cleared up.

SPECIAL CONDITIONS

Glossary

Abdomen	Area at the front of the body between the chest and pelvis.
Acupuncture	Therapy involving the insertion of needles into the body at determined points.
Acute	Of sudden onset and short duration.
Adrenaline	Hormone that stimulates the body in preparation for physical exertion, or when under stress.
Alexander technique	System of training to correct poor posture.
Allergy	Individual over-reaction by the immune system to certain harmless substances.
Ankylosing spondylitis	Inflammatory spinal disease that leads to vertebrae fusing together.
Annulus fibrosus	Outer fibrous layers of spinal discs.
Arthritis	Inflammation of one or more joints.
Carpal tunnel syndrome	Irritation of a nerve in the wrist.
Cartilage	Hard, smooth tissue covering the ends of bones to enable them to slide over each other.
Cervical	Of, or relating to, the neck (also the neck of the womb).
Cervical rib syndrome	Irritation of nerves at the base of the neck.
Chiropractor	Therapist whose approach to treatment involves manipulation of the spinal joints.
Chronic	Of long duration.
Coccyx	Small tailbone at the lower tip of the sacrum.
Diagnosis	Identification of a medical condition from its history, signs and symptoms.
Diagnostic picture	Broader view of diagnosis including the whole person, not just concentrating on the disease.
Diaphragm	Main muscle used in breathing, situated between the thorax and the abdomen.
Discs	Flexible structures between the vertebrae.
Facet joints	Pair of small joints connecting the vertebrae.
Fibrosis	Stringy and inelastic muscular state, caused by prolonged contraction.
Hamstrings	Group of muscles at the back of the thigh.
Herniation	Protrusion of pulpy disc material through the outer fibrous layers.
Hip Flexor	Muscle running through the pelvis, between the lumbar spine and thigh bone, that bends the hip.
Hormones	Chemicals secreted by certain glands in the body to regulate the function of other tissues.

Inflammation	Local reaction of the body to disease or injury, resulting in swelling, heat and pain.
Intervertebral	Between two vertebrae.
Irritation	Interference with a tissue that leads to symptoms or inflammation.
Joint	Junction between bones.
Kyphosis	Forward curve of the spine.
Ligament	Fibrous bands that hold bones together and stabilize joints.
Lordosis	Backwards curve of the spine.
Lumbago	Non-specific term for aching in the low back area.
Lumbar	Of, or relating to, the low back.
Manipulation	Use of the hands to move the body; commonly the 'clicking' of spinal joints to unlock them.
Massage	Use of the hands to relax and stretch soft tissues, especially muscles.
Metabolism	The chemical processes of the body.
Muscle	Tissue that contracts when stimulated by nerves.
Musculo-skeletal	Of, or relating to, the framework of the body – the muscles and the bones.
Nerve	Specialized collection of fibres that transmit signals between parts of the body.
Nucleus pulposus	Pulpy, inner core of a spinal disc.
Orthopaedic	Of, or relating to, the treatment and prevention of skeletal and muscular deformities.
Osteoarthritis	Degeneration of joints caused by wear and tear.
Osteochondritis	Temporary softening of bone and cartilage that alters the shape of vertebrae and results in stiffness.
Osteopathy	Holistic system of medicine that views each person individually and uses advanced manual skills in diagnosis and treatment.
Osteophytes	Small, abnormal projections of bone.
Osteoporosis	Thinning of texture and weakening of bone.
Pain-spasm-pain reflex	A vicious circle of pain, which causes spasm leading to more pain, and so on.
Pelvic tilt	Backwards rotation of the pelvis.
Pelvis	Girdle of bones at the lower end of the spine, joined to the legs at the hip joint.
Piriformis	Muscle between the sacrum and thigh bone located deep in the buttock.
Prognosis	Prediction of the course of an illness.

GLOSSARY

Prolapse	Severe herniation.
Psychotherapy	Treatment of mental or emotional disorders by psychological means.
Referred pain	Pain felt at a site other than the location of the problem.
Rheumatism	Non-specific name for general aches and pains in joints or muscles.
Rheumatoid arthritis	Disease causing inflammation of many joints.
Sacro-iliac joint	Joint each side of the sacrum, joining it to the main pelvic bone.
Sacrum	Triangular bone made of five vertebrae fused together, situated at the base of the spine.
Sciatica	Pain in the leg associated with low back pain; supposedly due to irritation of the sciatic nerve.
Scoliosis	Sideways curve of the spine.
Segment	Small section of the spine, based on one vertebra.
Sequestrum	Fragment of disc remaining in the spinal canal after herniation.
Spasm	Extremely hard, involuntary contraction of a muscle.
Spinal canal	Hollow section running along the length of the spine that contains the spinal cord.
Spinal cord	Collection of nerves that run along the spine between the brain and the rest of the body.
Spondylarthrosis	Arthritis of the spinal facet joints.
Spondylolisthesis	Forward displacement of one vertebra on another.
Spondylosis	Degenerative changes in the spine.
Subconscious	Of, or relating to, mental processes, actions or emotions that are not under conscious control.
Symptom	Feeling or sign that something is wrong.
Syndrome	Collection of symptoms that tend to occur together.
Synovial fluid	Fluid that lubricates and nourishes joints.
Tension	Tightness or overcontraction of muscles; inability to relax or unwind.
Therapist	Person who helps to resolve problems.
Thorax	Compartment of the body enclosed by the ribs; area between neck and low back.
Tissues	Collection of cells of a similar type that make up different structures of the body.
Trauma	Damage or injury.
Vascular	Of, or relating to, blood vessels.
Vertebra	One of the bones that make up the spine.
Visceral	Of, or relating to, the internal organs.
Whiplash	High speed trauma to the neck.

Index